Contents

Foreword

This book describes a journey in pursuit of understanding with the author cast in the role of everyman or, more precisely, every-general-practitioner. It is illuminated throughout by his delight in different forms and ways of knowing. He begins with a single consultation and proceeds via an authoritative analysis of the claims of contemporary evidence-based medicine to revel first in the naturalistic intellectual tradition and then, with palpably mounting excitement, the new insights which are generated by an understanding of chaos and complexity theory. He shows that each way of knowing has the capacity to inform and enrich the others and that none can lay claim to any sort of exclusive truth.

In 1998, I had the privilege of accompanying Kieran on a very small part of his journey. By chance, we both attended an extraordinary conference in Durham with the slightly less than seductive title of 'Advancing methodology in general practice research'. It had been organised by Frances Griffiths on behalf of NoReN, the Northern Primary Care Research Network, and it included a revelatory presentation by the sociologist David Byrne outlining the rudiments of chaos and complexity theory. Kieran and I found that this resonated so powerfully with our intuitive and experiential knowledge of general practice that, I think, neither of us ever felt quite the same again about the work that we do everyday. It suddenly made sense of why guidelines are of such limited usefulness in the reality of daily practice, why the same treatment applied to apparently similar people carrying the same biomedical diagnosis can have such very different outcomes and why the 'rolling out' of pilot initiatives is almost always disappointing. It opened up whole new areas of understanding and Kieran went on to use complexity theory as the intellectual basis of his future research. This book is a large part of the result.

More than 30 years ago, the American teacher and literary critic, Lionel Trilling, wrote about the distinction between sincerity and authenticity. Sincerity is the notion of being true to oneself through the achievement of a consistency between thinking, feeling and doing, whereas authenticity poses an even greater challenge because it recognises the existence of many, and potentially conflicting, selves which must be acknowledged and accommodated. In his introduction to *Ulysses*, Declan Kibberd sees the success of James Joyce as the realisation of authenticity. In the same way, Kieran Sweeney seeks, perhaps, to move beyond the traditional sincerity of John Berger's *Fortunate Man* and to explore the possibility of authenticity within contemporary general practice.

In *Ulysses*, James Joyce showed that the detail and complexity of a single day in the life of a single individual contains within it the breadth, depth and extent of the totality of human experience. Similarly, Kieran Sweeney finds all the fascination and challenge of general practice within a single consultation. Declan Kibberd writes:

Man's littleness is seen, finally, to be the inevitable condition of his greatness. What one man does in a single day is infinitesimal, but it is nonetheless infinitely important that he do it.

What happens between a patient and a general practitioner within a single consultation is also infinitesimal but nonetheless infinitely important. The tragedy is how poorly this is understood by those in power.

Iona Heath
April 2006

About the author

Kieran Sweeney holds arts and medical degrees from Glasgow University, a research Masters degree from Exeter University and a doctorate in medicine from the Peninsula Medical School, Universities of Plymouth and Exeter. He has been awarded honorary fellowships of the Royal College of General Practitioners and the Royal Society of Arts, and the Eric Elder Medal by the Royal New Zealand College of General Practitioners. After completing his medical undergraduate training, he completed an extended general practice training programme in the south-west of England, Paris and Brittany. He works as a general practitioner in Exeter (in the sixth doctor–nurse partnership in the NHS), as an Honorary Senior Lecturer at the Peninsula Medical School, and as Director of Research Management and Governance for the south-west peninsula. He acts as spokesperson for the NHS Alliance on Policy and Leadership.

Between 2000 and 2004 he worked for the Commission for Health Improvement, as part of the development team which devised the assessment framework for primary care organisations. He co-managed the first such assessment in Norfolk. Between 2003 and 2004 he was seconded to the Transition Team, which was established in order to set up the Commission for Healthcare Audit and Inspection (now the Healthcare Commission). After its establishment, he worked briefly as Policy Manager for Primary Care at the Healthcare Commission. He resigned from the Commission to start up a completely new general practice in Exeter in the autumn of 2004.

Kieran is a former Harkness Fellow and Visiting Scholar at the University of Washington, and during the mid-1990s he was a contributing health correspondent for *The Times* in London. He is a member of the Health Complexity Group, a collection of healthcare researchers, practitioners and philosophers who are examining how insights from the complexity sciences might help to explain the process of change in healthcare organisations. He has published around 100 articles, an Occasional Paper for the Royal College of General Practitioners, and seven chapters in various textbooks. He has produced three books. *The Human Effect in Medicine: Theory, Research and Practice* and *A Practical Guide to PCGs and Trusts* were both produced in collaboration with GP colleague Mike Dixon. *Complexity and Healthcare: an Introduction,* which he co-edited with Dr Frances Griffiths, was published by Radcliffe Medical Press in 2002.

Kieran recently received a personal commendation from the Honourable Annette King, MP, Minister of Health for the Government of New Zealand, for his contributions to the annual conference of the Royal New Zealand College of General Practitioners.

He is married to Barbara, a hospital business manager, and has four children.

Introduction

General practitioners are generalists. Most general practitioners understand that claim in the technical sense – they are unique among healthcare professionals in having diagnostic and management skills that transcend the arbitrary boundaries of specialisms. Compared with the breadth of clinical problems that general practitioners encounter, specialists are clinical partialists, addressing the parts, and only those parts, which their specialism can reach. The diabetic retina, the ischaemic foot, the menorrhagic uterus and the arthritic hallux are all meat and bone to the general practitioner's morning surgeries. Technical generalism is the bedrock of competent general practice.

But the generalism that primary care doctors encounter and explore is much wider than this. They have to understand the demands of contextual generalism, where the dynamic of a consultation undergoes a sea change, usually oscillating from the biomedical to the biographical, and sometimes – dizzyingly – back again. I start Chapter 1 by describing a consultation where precisely this happened, reminding us of the need to regard the biographical narrative as dignified, legitimate and grave, with all its attendant frailties, contradictions and post-hoc rationalisations. For the generalist, understanding context doesn't just mean knowing where the patient lives and how long ago she was divorced. It means accepting that the flow of a consultation may be determined by these very facts, in a way that prejudices and confronts the arithmetical acrobatics of biomedicine.

Yet we can take generalism a step further still. Implied by this second dimension of generalism – contextual generalism – is a fundamental shift in the type of knowledge upon which the consultation comes to be predicated. When we shift from biomedical to biographical perspective, we have implicitly accepted a shift in evidentiary framework, from scientific evidence to narrative evidence. This is the basis for a third dimension of generalism – evidentiary generalism. This term implies that, in practice, generalists have to feel comfortable swapping paradigms, deploying a range of world-views – the scientific, the narrative – in order to make sense of the reckless non-sense and wilful destruction of debilitating illness.

The purpose of this book is to reflect on the challenges concealed in this brief apologia for generalism. The book simply asks some questions about the questions that doctors ask. In Chapter 1, it asks why we need to bother with this exercise anyway, exploring what an explanatory model is, and why the conventionally accepted and hegemonic explanatory model in medicine should be scrutinised in the first place. And, as seems only right and proper for a book on general practice, it starts with the report of a consultation.

If Chapter 1 takes the first step of justifying why we need to ask questions about the questions that doctors ask, Chapter 2 leads us down the first pathway, tracing the intellectual origins of the scientific basis of clinical medicine. 'Why do doctors think the way they do?' is the question that is asked in this chapter. Chapter 3 takes us deeper into a critique of the scientific model in medicine, by interrogating its contemporary manifestation in the shape of evidence-based medicine. The aim is not to dispute, or to render disreputable, the notion of evidence-based practice. This would be foolish, and the chapter carefully presents the benefits to patients of this systematic approach to clinical evidence. Rather, the aim is to help us to think more about the way doctors think, and to introduce the notion that we 'think' in different ways. We 'know' things in different ways, too. This is what Chapter 4 deals with, tracing as it does the origins of the naturalistic enquiry, which has borne among its fruit the principles of qualitative research. The argument at this stage is as follows. We know things in medicine mainly from the perspective of medical science. The intellectual tradition of science in medicine is glorious, its contribution is immeasurably beneficial and its progress is magnificent. Yet it remains but one way of knowing – an explanatory model predicated on an epistemological framework of the scientific experiment, which in turn reflects a positivist ontology. Another way of knowing, which derives from the naturalistic tradition, draws on another type of evidence, often (but not exclusively) narrative evidence, and this epistemology reflects a more socially constructed ontology.

Chapter 5 introduces us to a third intellectual tradition, a third way of knowing. Reflecting on the fact that, in the light of advances, principally in mathematics and biology, many of the 'hard' sciences revisited and modified their explanatory models, this chapter traces the history of chaos and complexity. The description of its principles continues in Chapter 6, where examples of the application of complexity in commerce and economics as well as in clinical medicine are set out. Chapter 7 presents some practical examples of a methodology which draws on the principles of complexity to show how qualitative data can be re-explored, at a second-level analysis, if you like. The final chapter speculates on what all this can mean for the general practitioner. Is complexity the answer to life, the universe and everything? Read on to find out.

Chapter 1

Why bother? The need to understand explanatory models

A single consultation started the train of thought which has led to this book.

Some years ago, our practice nurse asked me to see Mrs B, an 85-year-old widow who as I recall, at the time of consultation, had been registered as a patient with me for about 15 years. I knew her well. Her husband, a pleasant chap who had been a builder, had died 5 years previously. Mrs B was pretty much estranged from her two grown-up sons, who were recurrent petty criminals, both serving prison sentences at the time of the consultation. Box 1.1 shows the conditions from which Mrs B suffered, and Box 1.2 shows her test results, which the nurse wanted me to review with her.

Box 1.1 Mrs B's comorbidity

Diabetes
Hypertension
Osteoarthritis
Macular degeneration
Hallux valgus

Box 1.2 Mrs B's test results

Glycosylated haemoglobin	9.7%
Blood pressure	180/96 mmHg
Total cholesterol	8.0 mmol/l
Body mass index	29 kg/m^2

Mrs B is not unusual, and my guess is that many people reading this book will know patients like her. When we met, at the practice nurse's request, I rehearsed the abundant evidence supporting interventions to lower her blood pressure, to improve the control of her diabetes and to reduce her lipid levels. I remember even thinking where the reference for this all lay (with a resumé in *Clinical Evidence*). I confess to feeling just a shade confident as I explained the abnormalities and how we could 'help' to reduce her risk. After a few moments I stopped – resting my case, as a barrister might say.

Mrs B remained silent for a moment or two. Then she said, 'Well, Jack's dead and the boys have gone.'

This has remained one of the most privileged communications I have ever received. As she delivered her words I sensed that she was saying something very profound, although its full implications eluded me for a number of years. Certainly on the day, the consultation changed tack and, looking back, we muddled through with a compromise strategy, and agreed to review the situation later. As Mrs B left, I sensed that the balance of influence in the consultation had rested firmly with her.

Analysing the consultation: 'Jack's dead, and the boys have gone'

This is really the pivotal sentence, out of which many of the concerns explored in this book arose. At the simplest level, one can say that the consultation, at the point when Mrs B made this contribution, moved from being doctor centred to being patient centred. It moved, one could say, from the biomedical domain to the biographical domain, or from clinical, evidence-based medicine to a consultation predicated on narrative-based evidence. But the shift was profound. When the consultation moved from its biomedical phase, it shed its parameters of *P*-values, absolute risk and numbers needed to treat. These were replaced by the parameters of the biographical phase of the consultation – led by Mrs B. Here despair, hopelessness, regret, guilt perhaps, and defeat were the parameters. Physical parameters had been replaced by metaphysical ones – two intellectual worlds seemed to have collided.

It is clear that, when Mrs B offered her contribution, the consultation took off in another direction. Up until that point, a fairly straightforward consultation was proceeding, drawing on scientific evidence gleaned from good clinical trials, many of them randomised and controlled, in the great tradition of scientific medicine. The remainder of the consultation, led by Mrs B, had nothing to do with that way of thinking, and arose from her lived experience. Yet in that context Mrs B's narrative evidence had more impact on the outcome of the interaction between Mrs B and myself than the clinical evidence-based observations with which I led the consultation. There were, one could argue, two ways of explaining things which were competing for influence – two explanatory models which at first sight did not seem to overlap much. At a deeper level, there were two types of knowledge jostling for influence. Two different ways of viewing and making sense of the world were at stake. But what constituted these three levels of understanding? This is what this book tries to explore.

Explanatory models, types of knowledge and world-views

Why bother? Why interrogate the explanatory model in medicine? An explanatory model provides a framework from which one can explore the receptive context within which professionals and patients conduct their conversations during consultations. Its propositions create boundaries within which these conversations can take place and also, in so doing, create constraints. For example, the postulates of homeopathy do not conventionally feature in these conversations, because they are not supported by the paradigm within which the current explanatory model in medicine is located. However, to describe medicine's explanatory model adequately, one needs to consider the world-view upon which it is based, and the type of knowledge constructed to populate and make sense of that world-view. Let me try to clarify succinctly the proposition that I want to explore.

The nature of an explanatory model, I argue, betrays a predilection for a certain type of knowledge – the collection of 'facts' which populate one's explanatory model. Medicine's conventional explanatory model is based on the scientific tradition. It populates that model with 'facts' arising from that tradition, in the shape of the results of scientific experiments, among which, for clinical medicine, the randomised controlled trial stands at the pinnacle. That preference, for one type of model over another, expresses the world-view that underpins the explanatory model. For medicine, I propose that the basis of the world-view underpinning that model is scientific positivism.

Before going any further, let me clarify some terminology and some initial standpoints.

I am using the term 'explanatory model' in a pretty straightforward, dictionary-based way. Thus I am taking 'model' to mean a set of postulates which serves to represent an entity that cannot be observed, and 'explanation' (similarly derived) to indicate the process of arriving at a mutual understanding or reconciliation (Kirkpatrick, 1994). In the context of this book, then, an explanatory model in medicine consists of a series of sense-making postulates that are located within the contemporary medical paradigm (using that term in its original Kuhnsian sense) (Kuhn, 1970). I am arguing from the viewpoint that the contemporary explanatory model in medicine is dominated by science – that is, science occupies a hegemonic role in that model. This is what I want to explore and reconsider.

In this book I will use the term 'science' as Chalmers (1982) does, in what he calls the 'widely held common-sense view of science.' Chalmers states:

> *Scientific knowledge is proven knowledge. Scientific theories are derived in some rigorous way from the facts of experience acquired by observation and experiment. Science is based upon what we can hear, see and touch. Science is objective. Scientific knowledge is reliable knowledge because it is objectively proven knowledge.*

This is similar to the way in which another philosopher of science, James Brown, uses the term 'normal science.' 'Most science,' Brown says, 'is normal science. It is what is done by all scientists who agree on the basics, that is what the world is made of, how things interact with it: normal science is a puzzle-solving activity' (Brown, 2001). Scientists, Brown goes on to say, work within a particular paradigm, or an accepted set of beliefs within a background of unquestioned theory. The scientific paradigm (Kuhn, 1970) involves some associative practices, including a basic agreement about ontology (what the world is made of) and epistemology (the nature of knowledge, its possible scope and general basis).

I can now put the central proposition of this book in slightly more formal, philosophical language. An explanatory model, one can say, is an expression of a particular epistemological standpoint, and this in turn reflects the ontological view held by the person who is supporting the model itself. An explanatory model is the product, if you like, of the interaction between the ontological view and the epistemological framework.

Science, in the sense that I have defined it above, accepts an objective singular rational reality that can be measured and verified. This associates science with positivism, first described by Comte (Honderich, 1995), by virtue of its acceptance of empiricism (all knowledge is based on sensory experience) and verificationism (if a statement is to be meaningful it must be empirically testable) (Brown, 2001). It also shares with positivism a sense of inexorability – of an inevitable progress inherent within scientific pursuit. And it shares with positivism a notion of hierarchy of knowledge, with knowledge derived from physics having the highest value. Scientific positivism is central to the ontological view held, usually more tacitly than explicitly, by those who support medicine's conventional explanatory model.

Thus defined, two characteristics are fundamental to science, namely linearity and reductionism. Linearity assumes a regular, proportionate and stable relationship between effect and antecedent cause. Reductionism refers to an approach to understanding phenomena by reducing the whole to its constituent parts, and assuming that the whole *is* the sum of its constituent parts. It is really important to hold these attributes of the scientific approach in mind, as I shall challenge medicine's explanatory model precisely at this level, by exploring another explanatory model (based on complexity) which emphasises the importance of interaction between parts, rather than reduction to parts.

In addition to the strict definitional issues, which it is important to get clear at the outset, it is also important to grasp the implications of this description of medicine's current explanatory model. By implication, 'science' as understood in this way is regarded as a purer form of understanding, where fact is considered more important than value and where explanation is confined to the expression of measurable and verifiable correlations between phenomena (Ruse, 1995). This is justified, I argue, because of the way in which the conception of science is embodied by the latest expression of the explanatory model in medicine, namely evidence-based medicine. Here evidence amounts to knowledge distilled from observation and experiment. These observations sit in a well-recognised hierarchy, with randomised controlled trials at the top, followed by partially or uncontrolled trials, with expert opinion very much at the lowest position in the league. The whole approach to evidence-based medicine, with its five steps – from defining the patient's problem to auditing one's performance in solving it – represents the puzzle-solving approach of normal science. And it makes clear assumptions, albeit tacitly, about the world and the practitioners who make sense of it, using the epistemological principles laid down by its most revered exponent, David Sackett.

In *Clinical Epidemiology: a Basic Science for Clinical Medicine*, Sackett and colleagues state 'the assumption is that medicine is rational and so are you' (Sackett *et al.*, 1985). Evidence-based medicine depicts a world that is rational and objective, and which can be measured empirically. In addition, it depicts a world in which experiments can be performed in closed systems where it is assumed that the researcher can stand outside the system, apart from it, manipulating one or two key variables in order to measure the outcome precisely. If in the course of this book this model is criticised, it is not to diminish the extent to which developments in science, which lies at the model's heart, have benefited mankind. Rather it is to place the role of science in the contemporary explanatory model in a wider context – a context in which, I shall argue, several different explanatory models are deployed, exchanged and accepted.

Now this use of the term 'science' is open to criticism. As it stands, it is strongly associated with the principle of induction, the process of generalising from a series of particulars. That argument is not logically justifiable (Chalmers, 1982; Honderich, 1995; Brown, 2001), nor are the issues of authority of scientific knowledge or Popper's falsificationism (Popper, 1963) accounted for. Nor, finally, is the issue of all observations being theory driven given proper accommodation (Polanyi, 1958). But the use of the term 'science' in this way is justified pragmatically. It accords with Chalmer's common-sense view of science (Chalmers, 1982) and Brown's definition of normal science (Brown, 2001), which are in themselves compatible with the way in which science is conceptualised in the current explanatory model in medicine (Sackett *et al.*, 1985).

Facing up to the evidence: chinks in the armour of the gold standard

Although 'O'-level Latin was still a prerequisite for entry to my medical school in Glasgow in the early 1970s, the training there was resolutely scientific. Bio-medical science was riding the crest of an intellectual wave (from which, as we shall see, it was to fall), doctors were held in indisputably high regard, and advances in technology, especially in the field of molecular sciences, held out the promise of dramatic new interventions which would conquer the most common fatal diseases affecting Western societies. It would be nearly two decades before the breathtaking manifesto of the Evidence-Based Medicine Working Group (1992) exhorted us to concentrate on assessing precisely what kind of (scientific) evidence we had available to address our clinical questions. To have questioned the medical model at that point would have appeared heretical (and stupid).

However, some tried. Ivan Illich introduced the notion of iatrogenesis, the process by which medical care itself could cause illness (Illich, 1975). Cartwright and Anderson (1981) published their seminal study of general practice patients not long afterwards, giving us the first hint that perhaps they were not so unthinking and passive as doctors assumed them to be. However, there was no real attempt to disarticulate the medical model, and the hegemony of science remained virtually impregnable up until the turn of the century.

I confess, along (I imagine) with many other healthcare professionals, to holding a fairly simplistic view of evidence during that time. The whole thing was rather a mystery really, but one took comfort from the fact that a randomised controlled trial was the best one could get, and one could pretty well bet one's life on the truth of their outcomes. The fact that many patients did, only to experience an unsatisfactory outcome, was one of the trends that led some practitioners to reappraise the nature of such trials, and to examine just how they were set up. The practice to which I belonged in the last two decades of the twentieth century did precisely that in relation to what appeared, to the untutored eye, to be a powerful body of evidence supporting the anticoagulation of patients who were suffering from atrial fibrillation. Around the time when this evidence was published, I had responsibility in my general practice partnership for clinical policies in this area. The publication of this evidence, authoritative reviews of it and policy documents based upon it had not been incorporated into our clinical practice. Although this could be seen as a simple oversight, excused by the bustle of daily general practice, my initial reading of the evidence led me first to articulate a more serious reluctance to incorporate the policy wholesale, and secondly to carry out a more in-depth review of the primary evidence. For me, the conclusion of this critique was the first step on the road to rethinking the whole model (Sweeney *et al.*, 1995). For this reason, the key points of the review are set out in the next section.

Warfarin and atrial fibrillation: a commentary from general practice

In 1992 the NHS Management Executive published a document which for the first time linked advice about commissioning services at the level of regional health authorities to contemporary clinical evidence (NHS Management Executive, 1992). I found one piece of guidance striking. In this particular section, the document advised those commissioning health services to link the provision of services for people with coronary heart disease to new evidence about the treatment of atrial fibrillation with the anticoagulant warfarin. My sense of failure upon reading this document was due to an instant recognition that this was not a policy that I was implementing in my own daily practice, nor was it a clinical policy in our practice as a whole. The sense of failure was magnified by our status as a training practice, where junior doctors passed through from time to time, relying on us – their trainers – to advise them about new developments. More importantly, we acted as an example of contemporary and exemplary general practice for them. Yet here was a policy that had already moved from the position of research reporting, through editorial comment in medical journals to the position of health policy in an executive document. All four partners in the practice, as it was then, held academic appointments. How could we have missed this new body of knowledge and consequently failed to act upon it? The solution seemed to be simple. Ascertain the evidence, build a clinical policy for the practice around that, audit our actions using the well-developed computer system that was already in use, and prepare to demonstrate the rapid change to our incumbent registrar.

Reviewing the evidence from the randomised controlled trials

In the early 1990s, six randomised controlled trials in Europe and North America produced results that supported the use of warfarin in both primary and secondary prevention of stroke in patients with non-rheumatic atrial fibrillation (Petersen *et al.*, 1989; Boston Area Anticoagulation Trial for Atrial Fibrillation Investigators, 1990; Connolly *et al.*, 1991; Stroke Prevention in Atrial Fibrillation Investigators, 1991; Ezekowitz *et al.*, 1992; European Atrial Fibrillation Study Group, 1993). Three trials also reported on the beneficial effect of aspirin compared with placebo. The design and results of these studies are summarised in Table 1.1 at the end of this chapter. The authors of the six primary prevention trials reported the findings of a collaborative meta-analysis of their results. The estimates of the reduction in relative risk of stroke with warfarin are shown for each trial separately in the right-hand column. Overall, these trials suggested that warfarin decreased the relative risk of stroke by 68%. The meta-analysis resolved other questions which had not been clearly answered by the individual trials.

Warfarin reduced the risk of both major and minor stroke, and was shown to be equally effective in men and women. The overall effect of aspirin was statistically significant but smaller. When data from both studies were combined, aspirin decreased the risk of stroke by 36%. Table 1.2 (at the end of this chapter) presents the results of these trials.

Within all of these trials the rate of serious complications from warfarin was remarkably low. In the meta-analysis the annual rate of cerebral haemorrhage was 0.3% in patients who had been treated with warfarin, and 0.1% in the control group. Taking these studies together, 40 patients with atrial fibrillation would have to be given an anticoagulant treatment for one year in order to prevent one stroke. Out of 1000 patients treated for one year, between 15 and 50 episodes of ischaemic stroke or systemic embolism would be avoided at a cost of between four and six measured episodes of bleeding over the same period.

Reviewing this evidence for general practice

On the face of it, the evidence from these trials suggested that a substantial benefit would be gained from using warfarin. Despite this, I together with my partners had been laggardly in applying this evidence. Early reading of one or two of the original studies provoked a series of questions about how reproducible these results might be in routine general practice in the UK. From this reading emerged the structure of a wider critique of the design and execution of this sextet of studies. In this critique, the salient questions about these studies concerned the participants in the trial, and the feasibility of reproducing the results in routine clinical practice.

- Were the characteristics of the populations that were studied comparable with the general population who may be offered this form of anticoagulation in primary care in the UK?
- Is the type of follow-up that was employed in these studies to ensure compliance feasible in day-to-day general practice?
- Is it possible to stratify risk and thus to individualise therapy in general practice?

The study populations in the atrial fibrillation trials

If the evidence from these trials was to be part of routine care for patients with this condition, we thought it was important to know the entry and exclusion criteria. In general these trials involved older patients, of mean age 69 years, about half of whom had hypertension and about a quarter of whom had angina. Around 20% had a history of heart failure and 14% were known to have diabetes. However, there was no standardisation between the trials with regard to the exclusion criteria. The rate at which patients were excluded from some of the trials surprised us, and made us reconsider the potential generalisability of the evidence. For example, in the SPINAF trial (Ezekowitz *et al.*, 1992) 93% of the eligible patients were excluded, of whom one-third had 'chronic alcoholism or a psychiatric or social condition rendering the patient unsuitable for anticoagulation.' A further 1600 patients were deemed ineligible for inclusion in the study, according to 'undefined administrative criteria.'

In the SPAF study (Stroke Prevention in Atrial Fibrillation Investigators, 1991) only 3% of a potential 18 000 eligible patients were entered into the warfarin arm of the study. Nearly 1000 patients in this study were excluded because the investigators could not be sure that they were followed up, and about 1700 patients refused to enter the trial once invited to do so. A separate list of exclusion criteria was applied to over 700 patients in the SPAF study, who were entered into the programme but not assigned to anticoagulant therapy. Of this group, one-third refused anticoagulant therapy and 6% were excluded because of 'repeated falls or unstable gait predisposing to head trauma.'

It began to look to us as if the patients who were entered into these trials represented a population with atrial fibrillation that was, to begin with, at low risk of bleeding on warfarin. They also seemed to constitute the population most likely to comply with the treatment and be amenable to follow-up. We checked the drop-out rates.

Despite the cautious entry criteria, quite large percentages of patients in all of the trials were withdrawn from warfarin therapy after entering the programmes. These included 38% of patients in the AFASAK study (Petersen *et al.*, 1989), 10% in the BAATAF study (Boston Area Anticoagulation Trial for Atrial Fibrillation Investigators, 1990), 26% in the CAFA study (Connolly *et al.*, 1991), 11% in the SPAF study (Stroke Prevention in Atrial Fibrillation Investigators, 1991), 31% in the SPINAF study (Ezekowitz *et al.*, 1992) and 21% in the EAFT study (European Atrial Fibrillation Study Group, 1993). The largest number of withdrawals was in the AFASAK trial, which was the closest to being a community study comparable with a UK primary care population.

Compliance and monitoring

Could the standard of care that these patients received be reproduced in routine general practice and achieve similar outcomes?

During the studies, patients were vigorously monitored in a hospital outpatient setting and underwent repeated physical examinations for the side-effects of warfarin treatment. The rigour of this follow-up programme did at least introduce the possibility that the perceived safety of the treatment, and in particular its low complication rates, was associated with the close medical monitoring of the patients who were receiving treatment. The concern among general practitioners in the UK was that such rigorous monitoring of patients was unlikely to be reproduced in routine clinical practice.

The clearest description of follow-up came from the Copenhagen AFASAK study, in which each patient had clinical check-ups twice in the first 6 months and every 6 months thereafter. Complete physical examination was undertaken, and echocardiography was performed to assess left atrial size. During the second year, echocardiography was repeated and the researchers obtained confirmatory evidence of continuing atrial fibrillation. Many of the other studies deployed similar rigorous clinical monitoring. The relevance of this to the problem of implementation was the difficulty of reproducing such rigorous monitoring, which was deemed sensible in the light of the potentially catastrophic side-effects of warfarin, the most serious of which is intra-cerebral haemorrhage.

Because of the potential side-effects of bleeding on warfarin, blood tests were performed frequently to ensure that the dose of warfarin was appropriate. In the trials that constituted the much cited body of evidence to support the use of warfarin in atrial fibrillation, blood tests were performed at monthly intervals, which probably fitted with the recognised schedule for monitoring in UK general practice. However, anticoagulant control and subsequent determination of the appropriate dose of warfarin were difficult, even in the hands of the experts who were conducting these trials. Table 1.2 at the end of this chapter shows the percentage of study days on which anticoagulant control fell outside the acceptable range, along with the annual rate of major bleeding episodes and the percentage of patients who reported minor episodes of bleeding on treatment. To our surprise, many of the trial patients were under-anticoagulated for a considerable proportion of time during the studies – nearly half of all the days on treatment in the CAFA study. Could this, we asked ourselves, be related to the low levels of serious bleeding that were observed in these trials?

Implications of this evidence for practice

There were conflicting views about the implications of this evidence for routine clinical care. Academic opinion, in the shape of editorials in well-respected journals, advised full and rapid implementation of the evidence (Laupacis, 1993; Lowe, 1993). However, routine clinical care seemed to be slow to catch up (Rassam, 1993).

On the basis of these studies, editorials in peer-reviewed journals encouraged doctors to consider giving anticoagulant therapy to patients with atrial fibrillation if there were no contraindications (Laupacis, 1993; Lowe, 1993). Some commentaries on the studies called for lifelong treatment, despite the fact that the mean duration of treatment in these trials was about 18 months (Laupacis, 1993). The results of these trials were brought to the attention of the NHS Management Executive, whose focus-group research identified anticoagulant treatment for patients with atrial fibrillation as a key element in purchasing negotiations for the then regional health authority corporate contract (NHS Management Executive, 1992). This was a crucial development. Here fresh research evidence was being linked to commissioning strategy at management level, despite a lack of vigorous reflection on the generalisability of these trials to routine clinical practice.

What did this review say about the nature of evidence?

Two important implications emerged from the publication of this review. This was the first time an extended appraisal of the components of a set of randomised controlled trials had been published.[1] It raised questions about the generalisability of scientific evidence, about the selection and exclusion criteria for trials and, emerging from these two points, concerns about how widely or safely this evidence could be incorporated into routine clinical care. In this respect it appeared to raise some questions about the model of evidence-based medicine, which was becoming an important influence at that time (Evidence-Based Medicine Working Group, 1992).

For me, it raised deeper questions. What was the basis of the randomised controlled trial, which had caused it to occupy pride of place in the hierarchy of scientific knowledge in medical practice? How and why had medicine come to

---

[1] The review paper was cited around 30 times in the next 5 years.

rely on the scientific paradigm, within which the randomised trial was one of the most powerful tools? These were questions about epistemology, about scientific positivism, and about the philosophical basis of research methods in general. A simple clinical query about the widely reported value of anticoagulation for this common cardiac dysrhythmia was leading us to ask basic questions about the scientific method.

To answer these questions, it seemed to be necessary to research the historical development of these ideas within clinical medicine. As we shall see, that intellectual journey simply led to more questions – about the origins of qualitative data, as opposed to the quantitative data of randomised controlled trials, and about the ways in which the other natural sciences were facing up to the massive paradigm challenges resulting from developments in mathematics and thermo-dynamics. My conclusion was bleak, namely that other sciences had assertively revisited their explanatory models, and some, including physics, had made sweeping changes to their understanding of the world. Medicine was yet to wake up to these challenges.

Table 1.1 Summary of randomised trials of warfarin and aspirin in patients with non-rheumatic atrial fibrillation

Study (year, country)	Design	Comparison	Setting	Duration (years)	Target	Person years of follow up	Annual event rate		% RRR of warfarin
							Placebo	Warfarin	
AFASAK (1989) Denmark (Petersen et al.)	Randomised Double blind Aspirin/Placebo	Warfarin, aspirin and placebo	OPD[a]	2.0	2.8-4.2 INR	398	4.8	1.4	71
BAATAF (1990) USA (Boston Area Trial)	Randomised Controlled Unblinded	Warfarin versus aspirin	OPD	2.3	1.2-1.5 PTR	435	2.9	0.4	86
CAFA (1991) Canada (Connolly et al.)	Randomised Double blind	Warfarin versus placebo	OPD[b]	2.5	2.0-3.0 INR	241	3.7	2.1	43
SPAF (1991) USA (Stroke prevention in atrial fibrillation)	Randomised Aspirin/Placebo Double blind	Warfarin versus placebo aspirin versus placebo	OPD	1.3	1.3-1.8 PTR	245	7.4	2.3	67
SPINAF (1992) USA (Ezekowitz et al.)	Randomised Placebo controlled Double blind	Warfarin versus placebo	OPD	1.7	1.2-1.5 PTR	483	4.3	0.9	79
EAFT (1993) Netherlands (European Atrial Fibrillation Study Group)	Randomised Secondary prevention trial	Warfarin versus aspirin versus placebo	OPD	2.3	2.5-4.0 INR	517	17.0	8.0	53

OPD = outpatient department; INR = international normalised ratio; PTR = prothrombin ratio; RRR=relative risk reduction.
[a] Echocardiography laboratory; [b] University centres.

Table 1.2 Percentage of study days where anticoagulant control fell outside stated range, annual rate of major bleeding episodes and percentage of patients with minor episodes

Study	% of days where INR/PTR		Bleeding episodes	
	Below lower limit	Above higher limit	Annual rate of major (%)	% of patients with minor
AFASAK	26	0.6	1.2	A
BAATAF	9	8	0.4	17.9
CAFA	40	17	2.5	16.0
SPAF	23	0.5	1.5	A
SPINAF	29	15	1.3	24.6
EAFT	32	9	2.8	20.9

INR = international normalised ratio; PTR = prothrombin ratio; A = Not reported.

Chapter 2

The biomedical tradition: why doctors think like doctors

Introduction

So why do doctors think like doctors? What kind of intellectual tradition has spawned the progeny of the biomedical model? To find out the answers to these questions, we need to go back to the origins of this approach in ancient Greece, and trace the development of that type of thinking up to the present day. This chapter presents a historical overview of the main influences that shaped and informed the current accepted medical model. It then looks at the current manifestation of that model, enshrined in the principles of evidence-based medicine (EBM) and, by presenting a brief critique of EBM, begins to unpick the features of a different, complementary way of thinking, whose intellectual pathway has yielded the principles of qualitative research. The next chapter explores that pathway in greater detail, defining its intellectual origins, and reflecting on what that means for the way in which doctors think in consultations.

Although this seems to be a helpful way of exploring how the contemporary medical model evolved, I accept that a pervasive weakness of historical accounts is that they are exposed to assumptions about the status of past knowledge. Such assumptions necessarily entail a degree of bias, through the interpretive prism of the historian. Thus they run the risk of conferring on past knowledge a degree of significance that it may not initially have had. So although historical accounts of medicine may not provide a perfect mirror of past events, they are useful for making explicit the assumptions that underpin the theory upon which the current accepted model rests.

The historical overview presented here is necessarily brief and eclectic, focusing on the principal contributors to our current understanding of the medical model. This historical overview will show that the twentieth century can be divided into two periods, the first one ending around the mid-1970s. Up until then, rational scientific progress in medicine seemed unstoppable, exciting discoveries peppered the medical landscape, and the status of the medical professions (at least in hospitals) seemed unassailable. However, by the last quarter of that century the supremacy of interventionist medicine was being called into question, and developments in mathematics, biology and computing were introducing the possibility of another paradigm applicable to the biological sciences, this time predicated on non-linear modelling rather than on the linear rationality of scientific positivism. I shall explore this paradigm in Chapter 5.

The origins of contemporary medicine: ancient Greece and the Dark Ages

Ancient Greece is generally regarded as the home of medicine, whose point of origin is commonly identified in the writings of the Hippocratic collection (Singer and Underwood, 1962; Porter, 1987; Greaves, 1996). Plato proposed a distinction between the healthy soul (in which reason occupied a superior position to passion) and organic social order, in which rational guardians possessed true authority (Porter, 1987). Dubos (1960) points out that Hippocrates' writings have had a biblical influence on the thinking that has underpinned medical practice throughout recorded history. According to Dubos, Hippocrates stands for rational concepts based on an objective knowledge of science in general, and of medicine in particular, liberating it from mystic and demonic influences (Dubos, 1960). There is an important identification here of the superiority of rationality and reason as conceived within positivism,[2] to the detriment of all that was seen to be irrational or non-rational.

Greek medicine had three fundamental characteristics that have contributed to its fundamental status in contemporary medicine. It had a unified theory of medicine (referred to as naturalism), it held an ontological view of diseases as specific and real entities awaiting discovery and classification, and it advocated an outlook based on empirical observation as a way of progressing knowledge (Greaves, 1996).

During the Roman period that followed, the second great medical name of ancient times, Galen, produced his writings. Their main contribution was to organise and restate systematically what had gone before, rather than to produce anything really new (Phillips, 1973). The prolonged period after Galen, from AD 200 to AD 1500, is still regarded as a regressive period for mankind in general, and medicine in particular – a view that is symbolised by the use of the term 'Dark Ages' to describe that era. Singer and Underwood (1962), for example, present the still widely held view of the Dark Ages of medicine as a 'period of progressive deterioration of the intellect', criticising medicine up to around AD 1500 mainly on the grounds of its lack of precise observation in anatomy and pathology.

The origins of contemporary medicine: Renaissance and Enlightenment

In contrast, the next three centuries, from 1500 to 1800, are projected in an altogether different way – the Renaissance and Enlightenment – in which medical progress was reawakened and medical theory and practice advanced. In the context of the history of medicine, the previous period of the Dark Ages was to be set aside, as an interruption to the inexorable progress of medical understanding which could be ignored (Cunningham, 1989). However, the same author (Cunningham, 1989) suggests that it was Hermann Boerhaave (1668–1738), a

---

[2] I use Brown's definition of positivism as predicated on empiricism (all knowledge is based on sensory experience) and verificationism (for a statement to be meaningful, it must be empirically testable) (Brown, 2001).

physician and teacher who lived in Leiden, who had a seminal influence on portraying (retrospectively) this progressive scientific view of medical history, which has continued to be widely held up to the present day:

> *In the early decades of the eighteenth century Boerhaave created a history whose peaks were Hippocrates, Bacon, Sydenham and Newton. Hippocrates first practised proper medicine, Bacon pointed out the means for its restoration, Sydenham effected its restoration into practice, and Newton provided the means to understand properly the working of the body.*

King (1982) has summarised the contributions of Francis Bacon (1561–1626) (to which we shall return in Chapter 4 on qualitative research) in his demand for precision in observation, and for repeated experimentation leading to cautious generalisation. The chief elements of the modern scientific method, King argues, are found clearly expressed in Bacon's writings. 'He recognised the need for controls', King writes, 'pointing out the dangers of hastily drawing conclusions, the need for verification and the return to particulars once the generalisation had been made.' Singer and Underwood (1962) argue that this huge influence ascribed to Bacon must be seen in the light of the achievements of the great Renaissance pioneer Andreas Vesalius (1514–1564). 'The masterpiece of Vesalius', they write, 'is not only the foundation of modern medicine as a science, but the first great positive achievement of science itself in modern times.'

The historical and intellectual link between Hippocrates, Vesalius and Bacon and Isaac Newton (1642–1727) now seems obvious to contemporary practitioners. Newton developed a physical system of science that claimed to be unified, absolute and objective. Medicine enthusiastically embraced the Newtonian ideal of this single schema, and each of its newly produced theories claimed to support and develop that ideal. In addition, Newton influenced modern medical thinking by developing the principles of mechanics, heralding a mechanistic model of science, populating the medical vocabulary with mechanical metaphors, and inexorably imbuing the medical model with linear thinking. The essence of the linear method was the acceptance of a proportional, steady, regular and predictable association between variables. Newton's approach was also reductionist, implying that phenomena could be described and hence understood by reducing the whole to its constituent parts and, more importantly, by assuming that the whole *was* the sum of its constituent parts. These parts were thought to be regulated by a small number of core laws, and were assumed to change in a smooth and predictable manner. With the adoption of these mechanical metaphors, a new discipline of iatrophysics (Greaves, 1996) emerged, which promoted the study of the body as a machine. Perhaps the most elegant application of Newtonian mechanics to clinical practice was the description of circulation by William Harvey (1578–1657) in 1628. Singer and Underwood (1962) strongly emphasise this important mechanical approach to medical practice and understanding exemplified by Harvey's description of circulation. 'The knowledge of the circulation of the blood has been the basis of the whole of modern physiology', they wrote, 'and with it the whole of modern rational medicine.' Greaves (1996) sees Harvey as rivalling Vesalius as the founder of modern scientific medicine. However, both can in part be accused of maintaining a rather solipsistic view of the rise of medicine in the West, by ignoring the staggering contribution to this field that was made by the Syrian physician

Ibn al-Nafis (1200–88), who described how oxygenation of the blood took place around 300 years earlier than anyone in Europe (Brown, 2001).

The last member of Boerhaave's heroic quartet was Thomas Sydenham (1624–1689), who practised in London between 1656 and 1689. His contribution to improving medical practice resulted from systematic observation of patients independently of any medical theory, and his focus on the typical manifestations of disease, rather than on a particular individual's unique experience of illness. Relying heavily on induction, his contribution was to derive general accounts from a multiplicity of individual case histories. Greaves (1996) argues that Sydenham had an ontological conception of disease, viewing diseases as real, distinct and natural entities that were awaiting discovery, ready to be allocated their pre-ordained position in a natural taxonomy. The conventional view of history sees Bacon, Harvey, Newton and Sydenham as key figures laying down the basis for the modern understanding of medicine and medical science.

The rise of science in medicine: the nineteenth century

The dawning of the nineteenth century marked an important watershed, not only in world politics (less than a quarter of a century had elapsed since the Declaration of Independence by the United States of America), but also for the rise of science in medicine. And it is perhaps fitting that scientific progress in medicine had its origins in Paris, when not just France but Europe in general was reeling from the consequences of the French Revolution of 1789–95. One of the consequences of the Revolution had been the removal of hospitals from the hands of the Church into those of the nation state. Medical politics, policies and institutions were vigorously reformed, and new programmes of medical enquiry and research practice were introduced by an enthusiastic and ambitious community of physicians based around Paris, where their salaried appointments gave them access to 20 000 beds in the city alone, outnumbering England's entire inpatient population at that time (Porter, 1997). The most significant change in clinical practice was the central role of the autopsy to corroborate bedside diagnoses. The tumours and infections that killed people became the focus of attention, and doctors were continually searching for correlates between clinical presentation and pathological lesion. Porter (1997) points out that early signs of this shift to a disease focus in medical practice had not exclusively occurred in Paris. The previous century had seen parallel traditions developing in Scotland and Germany in particular, and also in England – for example, through the contribution of Thomas Sydenham, whose work has already been mentioned.

Bichat (1771–1802) was probably the key influence in the Parisian movement at this time (Greaves, 1996). He emphasised the importance of anatomical dissection. 'Start cutting bodies open,' Bichat said, 'and hey presto, this obscurity will soon disappear' (quoted in Porter, 1997). It was ignorance of anatomy that had led physicians to neglect internal diseases. Before the rise in influence of physicians such as Bichat and his contemporary Corvisart (1755–1821), diagnosis had relied on the patient's history as well as clinical observation. However, although anatomy and the study of pathological lesions became dominant, clinical observation was not completely ignored. René Laennec (1781-1826) wrote an important treatise on the stethoscope (published in 1819), which encouraged physicians to bypass patients' accounts, thereby rendering diagnosis more 'objective.' Corvisart, Laennec and Bichat revelled in the amount of clinical material at their disposal in Parisian hospitals. Clinical medicine, Greaves (1996) argues, 'aimed to be a science, hinging on clinical detachment where empirical data were acquired through relentless examination of pathological lesions.' What this analysis implies is the increasing acceptance of reductionism in the medical explanatory model, expressed in the enthusiasm for anatomy to reveal the structure of the body, confident that, armed with this mechanical, Newtonian approach, an understanding of its function would follow.

Working alongside this cohort of clinicians, Pierre Louis (1787–1872) contributed significantly to the evolution of clinical science by advocating the use of numerical methods, using simple arithmetic to test the relative merits of competing therapies (Bynum and Porter, 1993). He encouraged clinicians to group together large batches of patients undergoing different treatments for the same condition, pointing out how differences in mortality would indicate the appropriateness of the chosen therapy. In doing this, it is clear that he paved the way for the clinical trial, whose randomised controlled form would emerge around 60 years later as the gold standard for evidence (Bynum and Porter, 1993).

Under the influence of the French, medical education across Europe and in America became more scientific and systematic. Foucault (1963) observes that this was 'the great break in the history of western medicine, dating precisely from the moment clinical experience became the anatomo-clinical gaze.' In Vienna, pathology dominated all other emerging medical specialties through the work of Rokitansky (Bynum and Porter, 1993). In England, Hunter occupied a similar privileged position to Bichat in Paris. The central position of anatomy in Edinburgh and London around the mid-point of the nineteenth century was highlighted by the gruesome activities of Burke and Hare, who first had the idea of selling dead bodies to anatomists (for £7 each), bypassing the grave (Porter, 1997). Their enthusiasm for the fees that such anatomical specimens could command led them to suffocate victims in preparation for their sale – murdering to dissect, as Wordsworth was later to observe.

This anatomical gaze, and the constant search for correlation with clinical abnormalities, was given a huge boost by refinements in optics, particularly the advances in microscopy that were introduced by Lister (1786–1869), the father of the more famous surgeon. This in turn had benefited from the brilliant lens-making capabilities of Carl Zeiss (1816–1888), among others (Bynum and Porter, 1993). It was in Germany that the new sciences of biology and histopathology were developed. The term 'histology' was coined in 1819, the year in which Laennec's treatise on the stethoscope was published.

Coming together (more by chance than by design) in Germany around the middle of the nineteenth century was the powerful triad of clinical ambition, technological advance, and financial support through the educational reforms of German rulers who invested heavily in academic science (Greaves, 1996). Understandings in physical chemistry helped physicians to interpret previously unfathomable physiological findings. A key figure in this domain was William Prout (1785–1850), who worked in England and was generally regarded as the father of biochemistry. Curiously, Prout's approach to clinical chemistry revealed one of the emerging tensions in the epistemological basis of scientific medicine. Prout was a vitalist, who believed that the chemistry of biological systems was something quite different from that of any physical system, being supported by what he called a 'vital force' (Brock, 1985, 1993).

Later in the nineteenth century, the attempt by Karl Ludwig (1816–1895) to debunk this mystic vitalism in physiological science did more than anything to root advances in this domain in quantitative positivistic and materialistic science. 'Every illness', Ludwig wrote in his *Textbook of Human Physiology* (cited in Porter, 1997), 'is a physiological experiment and each physiological experiment is an artificially produced illness.' By the late nineteenth century, technological advances had enabled scientists and clinicians to make the cell the focus of their research. These developments led to the crowning achievement of nineteenth-century medicine, namely the theory of contagionism and the germ theory of disease. This infection model, Ten Have (1990) asserts, 'turned out to be the most powerful paradigm of modern scientific medicine', singularly responsible for securing the decisive ascendancy of scientific positivism in medicine. The work of Pasteur and Koch is most closely identified with this domain, and although Koch's postulates were first published in 1891, they had in fact been described theoretically at least half a century earlier (Koch, 1891). Koch proposed that there were three essential elements in the ideal disease model, namely the causal agent, the pathological lesion and the clinical syndrome. It was, according to Greaves (1996), the most unambiguous expression of the dominance of scientific positivism in medicine, and it carried a series of important consequences and assumptions. Medical knowledge could henceforth only be determined by doctors, and progress would now only be linked to developments in science. Health was conceived as the absence of disease and 'illness' an imperfect account of it. Diseases existed as discrete real entities, with a universal nosology that was potentially completely discoverable (Wright and Treacher, 1982). Despite some swift modifications to the doctrine of specific causation (which was expanded to allow for more than one causal element), the rational and scientific basis of Koch's postulates has had an enduring influence on medical knowledge, practice and status ever since (Wright and Treacher, 1982).

Almost alone among contemporary commentators, Greaves (1996) identifies a weakness in the portrayal of Koch's postulates – in the way that they were portrayed as the triumph of positivism in medicine. Greaves asserts that the postulates essentially emphasise the primacy of the causal organism, but refer to it as if it were separate from the disease, in which case the other elements of the triad could take precedence, or occupy equal status with that of the causal organism. Virchow, who made a substantial contribution to the medical implications of cell biology by painting a picture of 'the republic of the cells', in which diseases were firmly situated in 'cellular abnormalities, multiplied through sequential divisions' (Virchow, 1858, cited in Porter, 1997), identified this confusion early on (Byron and Boyd, 1991). He described how 'the hopeless and never-ending confusion, in which ideas of being and causation have been arbitrarily thrown together, began when micro-organisms were finally discovered' (Virchow, 1895). What happened in practice, Greaves (1996) argues, was that the causal element was given primacy, but in so doing undermined the notion of objectivity, as a degree of judgement had been introduced into the concept of disease. In addition, the exercise of this judgement meant that the postulates in this 'ideal' model of disease were actually being used to construct the notion of disease, rather than to reveal a pre-existing (or even pre-ordained) notion of disease, which had been the original intention of the model. This attacked the very notion of value-free scientific knowledge as the source of medical understanding, but it did not diminish the importance of Koch's postulates in the progression of medical science in the twentieth century. However, its continued centrality to the medical model resulted from a complex interplay of social and political factors. The general optimism about human progress which characterised the nineteenth century and was captured, for example, in the writings of Comte and Mill (whom I shall discuss in greater detail in Chapter 4 on the origins of qualitative research), the desire to professionalise medicine (for example, through the Medical Act of 1858) and the statutory provision of healthcare, particularly in the area of public health and infectious disease (although the latter had been predicated on a quite different notion of infection called miasmatism; Singer and Underwood, 1962), all combined to sustain the centrality of the germ theory of disease in medicine and, more importantly, of the epistemological and ontological propositions on which that theory rested.

Porter (1997) summarises the progress of clinical medicine during the nineteenth century as follows: 'The pathological gaze penetrating the diseased body and the eye of microscopy formed part of the wider attempts to apply the methods of science to the whole medical enterprise, including the regular business of clinical medicine.' Advances in microscopy and optics led directly to the development of haematology as a medical specialty. Physiology was also supported by technical advances, and physiologists had achieved unprecedented influence, arguing that medical science had to understand the normal no less than the abnormal. The inexorable trend was towards objectifying findings accumulated at the bedside, and the monitoring of pulse, monitoring of temperature and serial measurements of chemical functions all became part of what was later to be called the 'work-up' of the patient. Clinical science itself became a byword for the advances of medical investigation that characterised the twentieth century. Huge advances in technology assisted developments in endocrinology and cardiology, and later assisted the introduction of two new specialties, namely genetics and immunology (Reiser, 1991; Devor, 1993).

This overview shows that science already occupied a hegemonic position in medicine by the end of the nineteenth century. A medical model was emerging which was firmly rooted in a positivist ontology – that is, a world-view that insists that anything which is measurable is real. Within this medical model, the body was regarded as a machine, the dominant metaphor was mechanical, and the relationship of antecedent cause to subsequent effect was regular, proportional and predictable.

However, the inexorable trend, first described by Boerhaave as an unassailable progression, does seem to have come together as a result of quite separate activities. Advances in strict biomedical understanding co-evolved with developments in optics, and both were helped by visionary political investments, such as the re-integration of hospitals into state control in France, and the huge investment in educational programmes in Germany in the early decades of the nineteenth century. And the triumph of rational scientific positivism in medicine, in the shape of Koch's postulates, is no longer seen to be as objective or intellectually celibate as was once thought.

Medicine in the twentieth century: an eclectic overview

Although it is impossible to describe each of the revolutionary innovations in scientific medicine that occurred during the course of the twentieth century, Table 2.1 shows a selection of the key achievements.

The application of scientific medicine to many diseases has been so successful that it is difficult to imagine what life must have been like during the epidemics of polio, diphtheria and whooping cough that ravaged society during the first half of the twentieth century.

Table 2.1 Selected milestones in medicine (adapted from Le Fanu, 1999)

Year	Achievement
1935	Introduction of sulphonamides
1941	Introduction of penicillin
1944	Development of kidney dialysis
1946	Developments in general anaesthesia (curare)
1948	First intra-ocular implant for cataract
1950	Streptomycin cure for tuberculosis
1954	Zeiss operating microscope
1957	Discovery of Factor VIII for haemophilia
1960	Development of the oral contraceptive pill
1967	First heart transplant
1969	Prenatal diagnosis of Down syndrome
1973	Introduction of the CAT scanner
1978	First test-tube baby
1979	Routine coronary angioplasty
1987	Thrombolysis for myocardial infarction
1996	Triple therapy for AIDS
1998	Sildenafil for the treatment of impotence
2003	First birth of a baby screened for genetic and therapeutic compatibility with sibling

Life expectancy has increased in developed countries, and medical interventions do appear to have contributed substantially to this (Bunker, 1995). There has been major progress in the field of antibiotic therapy, and in surgery, where advances in anaesthesia (particularly the introduction of the first heart–lung bypass machine in 1952 by John Gibbon) supported progress in heart surgery, leading to the first heart transplant at Groote Schuur Hospital by Christian Barnard (1922–2002) in 1967. Although it is beyond the scope of this book to present a systematic account of all the developments in scientific medicine that have taken place in the twentieth and twenty-first centuries, it would be a major omission not to mention the publication of the human genome map in 2002, hailed by the then American President Bill Clinton as the 'greatest discovery of mankind, something which will revolutionise the diagnosis of all diseases' (*Times*, 2002). The publication of this map represents the epitome of the reductionist approach, in which an understanding of function can be elicited from a detailed scrutiny of structure.

However, there is another side to the story. Despite the huge advances in scientific medicine, the number of acute serious illnesses in comparable groups of adults in the USA nearly tripled between the 1920s and the 1980s (Gillon and

Wesley, 1998). In 1974, the year before Ivan Illich published his seminal *Medical Nemesis* (Illich, 1975), a Senate investigation reported that approximately 2.4 million unnecessary operations were being performed per year in the USA at a cost of $3.9 billion and, more importantly, with a consequence of 11 900 deaths – more than the annual number of military deaths in Vietnam (Porter, 1997).

The analysis by Illich (1975) further fuelled this debate, arguing that conventional medicine had claimed a monopoly on the interpretation and management of health, well-being, suffering, disability, disease and death, ultimately to the detriment of health itself. Illich took the view that health broadly encompassed the processes of growing up, ageing, disease and death, using the coping mechanisms embedded in the culture and traditions of communities. Physicians, Illich argued, were now in the unenviable position of feeling that they had an *obligation* to make available any intervention which was available. There seemed to be an imperative among physicians to adopt a 'can do, will do' technological approach. Patients themselves began to register their dissatisfaction with what Skrabanek and McCormick (1989) later dubbed 'coercive healthism' by consulting alternative therapists, whose total number in the UK in the last quarter of the twentieth century was around 30 000, nearly equal to the total number of general practitioners (Le Fanu, 1999).

The dominance of the medical model predicated on science was called into question in the last quarter of the twentieth century by Engel's critique entitled *The need for a new medical model: a challenge for biomedicine* (Engel, 1977). Engel recognised that the science-based biomedical model was 'now the dominant model of disease in the western world' (Engel, 1977), and criticised it on three grounds, namely that it was reductionist, dualistic (disconnecting the body from the mind) and perfused the descriptions of bodily functions with mechanical metaphors. Although this model had a fairly wide folk appeal (Morris, 1998), it has suffered from confusion as to how the model addresses the notion of positivism and the role of science in medicine. In essence, in Engel's model the molecular phenomena remain firmly as the basis upon which the biological and social levels of reality are built. His analysis purports to give these levels equal weight, but he does not address the prerequisite elements at the core of medicine. Indeed he does not actually advocate that the psychosocial issues be placed at the centre of medicine, but only that they need to be *taken into account* (Puustinen, 2000). On the one hand Engel's position can be seen as subjecting psychological and social factors to scientific positivism, in which case any and all areas of life are vulnerable to medicalisation. On the other hand, the biopsychosocial model can be interpreted as a mechanism for excluding some areas from the domain of scientific positivism – but then one is left with the contentious decisions about which areas are, or are not, included within those realms. This confusion has never really been addressed, with the result that, although the model has never been actively opposed, its influence has been indirect at best and marginal at worst (Wulff, 1990; Morris, 1998).

Around the same time as Engel was advocating his new model, patients themselves developed a less meek and accepting role in the medical encounter, foregoing the assumption that doctors always know best and that patients do not really want to know what is wrong with them, because it might cause them anxiety. One English GP who was interviewed in the 1980s admitted that 'I find the older working classes and generally the lower middle classes of all ages easier to deal with than my own sort. My own sort ask complicated questions and are often dissatisfied with the answers' (Cartwright and Anderson, 1981).

A closer examination of the chronology of scientific discoveries in medicine during the twentieth century suggests that by the late 1970s many of the more spectacular discoveries had been made, and that from then onward there was a relative decline in major advances (Le Fanu, 1999). Even self-confidence within the profession itself has been damaged – for example, by the inability to contain the AIDS epidemic, and the confusion over the relationship between bovine spongiform encephalopathy (BSE) and Creutzfeldt–Jakob disease (CJD), which sparked further fears with regard to other potential pathogens introduced into the food chain as a result of ignorance.

The propriety and respect generously afforded to the medical profession throughout most of the twentieth century have been seriously damaged by the egregious and well-publicised failures of some prominent clinicians, most notably the cardiac surgeons in Bristol Royal Infirmary and the mass murderer Harold Shipman. Offering his predictions for the twenty-first century at the end of his vast tome, Porter concludes:

> *We have invested disproportionately in a form of medicine whose benefits often come late, which buy little time, and which are easily nullified by external, countervailing factors. Punitive interventionist medicine has played a modest part in shaping wider morbidity and mortality patterns within the community, and in terms of its professed aims – the greatest health of the greatest number – the Olympian verdict must be that much medicine has been off target.* (Porter, 1997)

Sir David Weatherall, Regius Professor of Medicine at Oxford (quoted in Porter, 1997) pointed to the root cause. 'The trouble is', Sir David observed, 'although we have learned more and more about the minutiae of how these diseases make patients sick, we have made little headway in determining why they arise in the first place.'

During the last quarter of the twentieth century, developments in fields that had not previously been directly related to medicine, such as computing, mathematics and ecology, began to inform a paradigm debate that was emerging within the medical profession (Kernick and Sweeney, 2001). This debate focused on observations provided by complexity theorists on a wide range of biological systems, which appeared to challenge the reductionist approach and linearity of the contemporary medical model. I shall explore the contribution of this field and its relevance to the medical model in Chapter 7.

Linearity in the National Health Service

The success of the scientific method extended well beyond the fields in which it originated. Drawing on the scientific paradigm, Adam Smith and David Ricardo advanced the laws of economic interaction (Fukuyama, 1993), and sociology and politics also tried to become sciences. This linear paradigm reached its zenith towards the middle of the twentieth century, when it was applied to modernisation theories of Third World development, international relations and public policy (Geyer, 2001).

It also influenced organisational development, not least in the thinking that underpinned the development of the National Health Service (NHS) in the UK. The machine metaphor for Newton's universe was translated into a desire to understand the structure and parts of all systems, and to build organisations on that basis. As early as 1911, Taylor published his theories of scientific management, with the underlying model of the organisation as a machine. The importance of mechanical metaphors in this explanatory model cannot be underestimated. Even up to the 1990s, these deeply embedded beliefs were expressed in the management predilection for re-engineering – a movement whose weaknesses were attributed to its failure to acknowledge the role of ordinary frail people in organisational life (Hammer, 1995).

In the UK, the NHS enthusiastically embraced this Taylorist approach, but only after an initial period, spanning its first 25 years, of management by diplomacy (Harrison, 1988). The command-and-control approach in the NHS, recalling the wartime circumstances in which hospitals were first brought under central control, is epitomised by the far-reaching Hospital Plan for England, which was devised in the 1960s but was not implemented for another decade (Department of Health, 1962). In the early 1970s, healthcare policy strategists agreed that the administration of the NHS was in need of an overhaul, but their solution, in the form of the *Grey Book* (Department of Health, 1972), testifies further to the confidence in linear, algorithmic solutions at that time. The *Grey Book* adopted a rigid, centralised approach to resolving the administrative confusion in the NHS. However, its insensitivity to local context exposed its inherent weaknesses almost as soon as its recommendations were implemented (Kember and MacPherson, 1994), and the structural reorganisation that it underpinned is generally viewed as a failure (Klein, 1989). The Thatcher reforms of the NHS, which were instigated after the review conducted at the then Prime Minister's request by Sir Roy Griffiths, demonstrate the extent to which strategy in healthcare was influenced by commercial business philosophy. In his much quoted comment in which he lamented the lack of managerial accountability, Griffiths wrote that 'If Florence Nightingale were carrying her lamp through the corridors of the NHS today, she would almost certainly be searching for the people in charge' (Department of Health and Social Security, 1983). Over a decade later, when Robinson and LeGrand (1994) evaluated another set of NHS reforms, they were unable to say whether the reforms had had a positive or negative impact. Hinting that the problems which were encountered as a result of the contemporary approach to healthcare strategy were more complex than had been envisaged, Robinson and LeGrand (1994) wrote that 'There are rarely simple answers to simple questions, usually because the questions are not actually simple.'

Summary

The general picture painted in this overview follows a widely accepted view of the history of medicine which characterises medical developments as involving a continuous, inexorable rise in the understanding of science, predicated on a rationalist positivist ontology. The evidence to support this picture is substantial, and while open to the considerations discussed above, it has helped to shape the view that the dominant biomedical explanatory model is predicated fundamentally on a reductionist conception of disease, in which the body acts as a machine, with disease events proceeding in a linear way through a sequence of measurable, regular and predictable causes and effects (Morris, 1998). The way to understand a diseased state, according to this model, consists of a detailed scrutiny of the structure of that state, achieved by reducing the whole to its constituent parts, and assuming that the 'whole' of that diseased state was the sum of those parts. Moreover, drawing on Newtonian thinking, it is assumed that those parts interact in a regular and predictable way, from which generalities of the diseased state may be constructed.

Not all commentators agree with this view. Almost a lone voice, Greaves (1996) proposes that this view, whose central pillar is the notion of a predetermined thread leading to the current understanding, is in fact a post-hoc rationalisation, and that it is weakened at its very source, namely the germ theory proposed by Koch. Theorists explored the contribution of social and psychological factors (Engel, 1977) but, despite some intriguing evidence – presented in the medical profession's leading journals – that cultural factors seemed to play a part in determining physicians' and surgeons' own practice, the impact of Engel's expanded model remained modest (Brook *et al.*, 1988; Garratini and Garratini, 1993). Others, notably Le Fanu (1999), argue that the spectacular advances in medicine occurred across a rather narrow spectrum and were more prevalent in the first three-quarters of the twentieth century than in the last 20 to 30 years. The scientific paradigm influenced fields well beyond those in which it originally developed. Throughout its history the NHS has experienced a series of reforms, all of which demonstrate a linear, mechanical approach to organisational development, testifying to the influence of that paradigm.

Had the conventional biomedical model, by the late twentieth century, exhausted its repertoire of problems to address, as Plsek (2002) argues? How might the observations from the complexity sciences, which were becoming increasingly widely reported in the medical literature, affect the model? I shall return to these questions in Chapter 5. To take this argument further, I shall now look at the contemporary manifestation of the biomedical explanatory model, in the form of evidence-based medicine. This model currently constitutes the bedrock of clinical medicine, and its integration into mainstream clinical thinking has embedded a hierarchy of evidence into current clinical practice. The nature of this evidence, refined as it is in various forms, the purest of which is considered to be the randomised controlled trial, remains resolutely scientific.

But think again of Mrs B. 'Jack's dead', she exclaimed, 'and the boys have gone.' Her intervention was pivotal in that seminal consultation. What explanatory model was she deploying? Chapter 4, which traces the origins of the principles of what we now call qualitative research, addresses this question. First, however, I shall explore the current manifestation of the scientific method in clinical practice, in the form of evidence-based medicine.

Chapter 3

Evidence-based medicine: the contemporary manifestation of the explanatory model in medicine

Introduction

The overview of the historical rise of science in medicine that was presented in Chapter 2 supports the proposition that, in the nineteenth and twentieth centuries, science came to occupy a hegemonic position in the explanatory model in medicine.

There are certain important epistemological implications for that model, namely that it is predicated on rational positivism, with an ontological conception of disease as real and distinct entities awaiting discovery and classification. In this chapter, I shall dig deeper into the explanatory model by describing and critiquing its contemporary manifestation in the form of evidence-based medicine (EBM). The purpose here is to develop the argument that is unfolding in this book, from a justification of the proposition that science dominates the model to an exploration of the implications of that model for everyday general practice. The aim is to arrive at a position in the argument where it can appropriately be held that, although science is a necessary (and indeed vital) component of the explanatory model, it is insufficient in itself to constitute that model.

Let us recall what is meant by the term 'evidence-based medicine.' The method is described as having five steps (Evidence-Based Medicine Working Group, 1992; Oxman *et al.*, 1993; Davidoff *et al.*, 1995; Rosenberg and Donald, 1995; Dawes, 1996; Sackett *et al.*, 1996).

- A clear clinical question is formulated from the patient's presenting problem.
- A literature search is conducted in order to identify relevant published articles that consider the problem.
- The evidence is accessed and evaluated (or critically appraised).
- Valid and useful findings are implemented in clinical practice.
- An audit of performance is conducted.

The 'evidence' in EBM refers to a hierarchy in which the findings of fully randomised controlled trials are at the top, followed by less well-controlled trials, cohort studies, expert consensus views and authoritative opinion.

This chapter explores EBM in four stages. First, the principles of EBM are explained and placed in context (Dawes, 1996). Next, I reflect on a description of the method (Rosenberg and Donald, 1995) and an early example of its application in an acute medical unit of a teaching hospital (Ellis *et al.*, 1995), both of which were quite heavily criticised in the correspondence columns of the peer-reviewed journals in which they appeared. In the third section, I briefly explore how EBM has been integrated into the current framework of general practice. Finally, I pose the following question. How could patients in general practice benefit from EBM?

The principles of EBM

Right at the outset, the instigators of EBM claimed that it 'aimed to de-emphasise unsystematic clinical experience and intuition as sufficient grounds for taking decisions in clinical practice' (Evidence-Based Medicine Working Group, 1992). Rather, the appraisal of evidence from clinical research was to be seen as the evident and proper basis for clinical practice. The process through which EBM was to be applied seemed to be straightforward. Patients present with problems which are turned into clinical questions. The answers to these questions are then based on the best available evidence, which is obtained by searching for and critically appraising the relevant studies.

After this initial description was published, a series of articles in the *Journal of the American Medical Association* entitled the 'Users' guides to the medical literature' illustrated the principles of EBM in greater detail (Guyatt and Rennie, 1993; Guyatt *et al.*, 1994), and demonstrated the importance of four basic outcome statistics, namely risk ratios, relative risk reductions (the complement of the risk ratio expressed as a percentage), the calculation of absolute risk reduction, and finally the numbers needed to treat (the inverse of the absolute risk). These proved to be extremely helpful in clarifying evidence at the population level.

What, then, were the advantages to which the advocates of EBM wished to draw attention? First, it offered a better way of deciding which treatments or clinical approaches could be usefully incorporated into practice, and which should be discarded. In turn, this could inform better decisions with regard to commissioning and providing services. It also provided a common language for critical appraisal of new evidence, which in itself might encourage the design of better trials and provide a sounder basis for undergraduate and continuing postgraduate education.

EBM wasn't rocket science. Its principles could be shared by healthcare professionals from different backgrounds (including non-clinicians), and by lay people, at any stage of their careers (Rosenberg and Donald, 1995).

However, early on in the adoption of EBM, practical problems emerged. It was conservatively estimated that it would take two hours to focus on a clinical question and then find, appraise and act on the evidence (Rosenberg and Donald, 1995). To do this, one would require access both to the appropriate computer software and to the Internet. Although it wasn't difficult, it took time to acquire the skills necessary to practise EBM properly. A plethora of protocols, guidelines and clinical synopses was produced to address these practical teething problems (Dawes, 1996).

Applications

Within three years of the publication of the principles of EBM, two seminal examples of its application in clinical practice in the NHS were published, one in secondary care and the other in primary care (Ellis *et al.*, 1995; Gill *et al.*, 1996). In the former example, over 100 acute medical admissions were studied in order to ascertain how many of the treatments that had been offered to the patients were evidence based. Around 82% of the patients were judged to have received evidence-based interventions; 53% had received interventions supported by one or more randomised controlled trials, and 29% were offered interventions that had been unanimously judged to be supported by convincing non-experimental evidence. Similar estimates were obtained in a study of two days of consecutive consultations in general practice (Gill *et al.*, 1996). Around 81% of the patients in this study received interventions that were either supported by one or more randomised controlled trials or were supported by convincing non-experimental evidence.

Thus EBM seemed to represent the pinnacle of the scientific tradition underpinning clinical medicine. It embedded a hierarchy of evidence, encouraged critical appraisal to distinguish between good and poor evidence and, with its clear explication of the concepts of absolute and relative risk, it made a major contribution to increasing our understanding of population-based evidence. How, then, could it attract the substantial body of criticism that it did? Many of the critiques focused on a central issue. Doctors don't practise medicine in populations – they consult face to face with individuals. Let us now briefly consider the gist of these objections.

Reservations

Iggo (1995) and Charlton (1995a) both challenged EBM on the basis of its central strength, namely the robustness of the evidence that forms its basis: 'a major fault with evidence-based medicine is its emphasis on randomised controlled trials' (Iggo). The results of such trials cannot be easily extrapolated to a particular target group, they argued, without taking into account relevant *contextual* knowledge.

Some critics, such as Fowler (1995), were clearly angered by some of its claims. 'Evidence-based medicine', argued Fowler, 'is a neologism for informed decision making . . . the presumption is made that the practice of medicine was previously based on a direct communication with God or by tossing a coin.' Other critics (Bradley and Field, 1995) of the paper by Gill *et al.* (1996) argued that assignment of diagnoses in the study achieved a reduction in complexity of management at the cost of 'drifting from the reality of many patients presenting with more than one problem.' And, they asked, 'what about people who did not have a diagnosis?'

One of the most enduring criticisms of the model accused it of measuring only what is measurable: 'There are no suggestions on how practice relating to unmeasurable aspects is to be guided' (Smith, 1995). And Bradley and Field (1995) stated that: 'Not all that is measured is of value, and not all that is of value can be measured.'

One of the key claims repeatedly made by proponents of EBM was that it constituted a new paradigm (Evidence-Based Medicine Working Group, 1992; Sackett *et al.*, 1996). It is important to look at this claim in some detail as, if substantiated, it would have serious implications for the unfolding of a new chapter in the epistemological evolution of biomedicine. Was the claim justified?

The claim that EBM constituted a new paradigm

Kuhn (1970) uses the term 'paradigm' to describe a set of shared assumptions or received beliefs in a scientific community. His central thesis is that groups of scientists imagine, think and research within a clearly defined set of assumptions which define the possibilities and also the limits of their endeavours. They use a technical language that encompasses a core group of theories, and then occupy themselves largely by solving only those problems that this technical language can express. Only when the need to answer questions that cannot be dealt with within the assumptions of a current paradigm becomes pressing can the assumptions be seriously challenged. Kuhn (1970) suggests that it is at (rare) times like these that new paradigms appear. He describes their appearance as 'a reconstruction of the field from new fundamentals, a reconstruction that changes some of the most elementary theoretical generalisations.'

Judged against these two criteria, one cannot confidently support the proposition that EBM constituted a new paradigm. First, its conceptual origins go much further back than the key synthesis of EBM thinking, *Clinical Epidemiology: a Basic Science for Clinical Medicine* (Sackett *et al.*, 1985). In the last chapter I referred to the work of Pierre Louis in Paris in the 1830s, who developed the first firm epidemiological approach to clinical thinking by comparing the outcomes in two populations of patients who were offered different treatments (Lilienfield and Lilienfield, 1979). Clinical epidemiologists had been working with evidence-based approaches for much of the twentieth century (Armenian and Lilienfield, 1994), and in the 25 years or so preceding the publication of the EBM manifesto (Evidence-Based Medicine Working Group, 1992), the number of published randomised controlled trials – mainly in secondary care, but increasingly in primary care – increased exponentially (Silagy and Jewell, 1994). Case–control methods and statistical techniques were developed throughout the first half of the century as sociologists began to tackle health problems as social issues (Lilienfield and Stolley, 1994). Doll and Hill (1950) were clearly publishing the best available evidence when in 1950 they reported one of the first studies linking smoking and lung cancer. In a seminal overview of medical research, the pivotal importance of randomised controlled trials was championed by Cochrane (1971), who described them as a 'beautiful technique of wide applicability.'

Secondly, before the EBM protagonists laid out their position, others had laid claim to introducing a paradigm shift. In theoretical terms, one could argue that McWhinney (1983) had a stronger case. As we saw in the previous chapter, he was one among a range of commentators who appeared to be reconsidering the explanatory model in medicine. In the clinical paradigm that was presented in the historical overview, disease was viewed 'objectively', independently from the person who was suffering from it. Mind and body were considered separately, each with their own diseases. In the early 1980s, McWhinney outlined what he claimed constituted a new paradigm which defined a view of medicine that 'would emphasise the patient, the doctor–patient relationship, and the language of illness' (McWhinney, 1983). Indeed, on a more muted level, the Royal College of General Practitioners (1972) had been supporting this model as one of the principles underpinning its vocational training.

The notion of evidence-based diagnosis

However, it is within the notion of diagnosis that the epistemological preferences of the EBM model are most interestingly revealed. In its first analytical step, EBM encourages us to define a clear clinical question. Two implications follow from this. First, if there is no clear clinical question, the model does not apply. Those who support the model are clearly in agreement with this, and it is not intended to apply to those circumstances, thus excluding the substantial number of general practice consultations which proceed without a firm diagnostic label. Secondly, where there is a clinical question, the framing of that question betrays a preference for the type of knowledge that biomedical science can bring to bear on the issue. Take, as an example, one of the EBM diagnoses that was identified and explored in the key paper by Gill *et al.* (1996) from general practice. A patient presents with worry, insomnia, palpitations and poor appetite. If a 'diagnosis' of anxiety is made, the literature can be searched for randomised controlled trials of benzodiazepines, and an appropriate evidence-based treatment applied. What has happened is that those aspects of the issue that can be usefully collated to form a 'clinical' question, and only those aspects, are abstracted. In doing this one has tacitly expressed a preference for selecting out those elements of the issue that can possibly be illuminated by the type of knowledge which is constructed from the epistemological standpoint of the model, in this case randomised controlled trials. However, if in this patient's presentation one identifies a set of related contextual issues as important – for example, a background of grinding poverty, a poor marriage and estranged children – one could construct a different but equally relevant question. In doing this one would again tacitly be expressing a preference for the epistemological standpoint in which narrative knowledge was the accepted currency. One's gaze on the 'case' would have moved from the biomedical to the biographical, just as occurred during Mrs B's consultation described in Chapter 1. And, just as in her case, one could see the 'case' in metaphysical terms, exploring the issues of hopelessness, despair, guilt, shame and humiliation. Thus we can see that the EBM model sits as one way of gazing upon issues – an extremely well-developed and robust way, but not a unique analytical method. The analogy can be made with scientists exploring the nature of light. They can 'look' at light as it 'appears' in terms of photons and packets of energy, and they will learn a lot, but they will be completely oblivious to the wave properties of the same phenomenon.

Thus, in general terms, the concept of 'diagnosis' in general practice is broader than the strictly biomechanical diagnosis that is used in randomised controlled trials, the cornerstone of the edifice on which the claims of EBM are based. Patients most often present to their GPs not with diseases, but with illness stories consisting of a collection of unorganised symptoms and signs. The process of defining a disease from such an illness story is a selective and narrowing abstraction (Kleinman, 1988).

Making a diagnosis is often an evolutionary process. Definitive diagnoses (in this broad sense) may be made retrospectively or indeed not at all. Formulating a diagnosis in general practice can take weeks or months, and the exact moment when a diagnosis becomes 'clear' may be difficult to determine. Here the evidence suggested that the general practitioner uses time appropriately as a powerful diagnostic instrument (Balint, 1957). Often the general practitioner formulates a series of diagnostic 'hunches' early in the consultation, using clues from their background knowledge of the patient and perhaps of the patient's family (Elstein *et al.*, 1972). Often the practitioner is forced to bypass confident diagnosis and adopt a decision pathway that approximates to symptomatic treatment (Howie, 1972). Diagnoses are sometimes made retrospectively, when the treatment confirms the putative diagnosis. However, if antibiotics are given for a sore throat, the diagnosis of bacterial tonsillitis may be supported, but it is hardly confirmed.

Until recently, the way in which medical students were taught diagnostic skills reflected this predilection for the scientific method. Traditionally diagnosis is taught to medical students (at least initially) as though it were an inductive process. First the facts are gathered without the prejudice of preformed bias, and only then, when all of the relevant pieces of the jigsaw have been assembled, does the full pattern reveal itself. However, most clinical problem solving is better taught as hypothetico-deduction (Royal College of General Practitioners, 1972) or, putting the same idea more simply, 'guessing and testing' (Marinker, 1981). For general practitioners brought up in this tradition, the early years in practice involve a lot of 'unlearning' of approaches that have been acquired during medical school education (Marinker, 1970; Williamson *et al.*, 1979).

The evidence in EBM

EBM encourages the critical appraisal of the best available evidence in order to solve clinical problems (Sackett and Rosenberg, 1995). For the most part, the evidence referred to is found in the results of randomised controlled trials or is collated in systematic reviews or meta-analyses. In setting out the principles of EBM, its proponents argued very persuasively that the breadth and explanatory power of a randomised controlled trial are the cornerstone not only for EBM, but also for evidence-based public health, evidence-based hospital administration, evidence-based purchasing and evidence-based consumerism (Sackett and Cook, 1994).

Let us remind ourselves what, precisely, a randomised controlled trial involves. In a randomised controlled trial, a group of individuals – the study cohort – is identified by virtue of its members sharing a common characteristic – for example, a particular disease or risk factor. The researchers randomly allocate each member of the cohort to one or more study groups, each of which receives different interventions, preferably in a way that is not known to either the researcher or the subject – so-called 'blinded intervention.' After a period of time the outcome for each group is ascertained and the findings are compared. Thus randomised controlled trials aggregate the benefits and disadvantages of alternative interventions in comparable populations within the same experimental environment. The idea is to balance the populations, the intervention and the assessment process, so that the only difference distinguishing the two, at the end of the observation period, will be attributable to the intervention. The key issue for the clinician is to consider how that population-based outcome may be applied to the individual patient.

The problem for all clinicians when using the results of EBM is simply this. Faced with a patient's particular clinical problem, the doctor needs to know whether the outcome statistic from a relevant trial applies to *this* patient, in *this* consultation, in *this* particular environment. However, these vital questions cannot be answered. Outcome statistics reflect the *average* experience of each group, and extrapolation with precision from that group average to a particular patient's chances is impossible. An extrapolation can be made, matching the consulting patient's characteristics with those in any relevant study, but the accuracy of this extrapolation is a matter of degree. What can be judged is the average order of probability in a large group of people whose personal and disease characteristics bear a resemblance to those of the patient.

In a clinical trial, a group of patients who share the same diagnosis may exhibit quite different patterns of illness behaviour. They may exhibit different symptoms or experience differences in the severity or rate of progress of the subject condition. In randomised controlled trials, these individual experiences are grouped together for the sake of simplicity and clarity, and the results are summated results from the combined experiences of a heterogeneous population of individuals. Although the intention is to distribute potential biases equally between the two groups, this does not eliminate the biases – it just disperses them, albeit in a particular manner. In this sense, comparisons between the groups will be unbiased but they run the risk of conflating several causal processes. A second difficulty concerns the relevance of the data from the population in the trial to the situation of the individual patient in the consulting room. To find out the extent to which the results of a trial should apply to a particular patient, the doctor needs to know what kind of patients were in the trial.

This critique is not intended to diminish the contribution of the randomised controlled trial to the clinical care of patients. Some of the simplest interventions have been subjected to this kind of trial. A classic example is the use of aspirin in secondary prevention of ischaemic heart disease (Second International Study of Infarct Survival Collaborative Group, 1988), trials of which have resulted in subsequent worldwide benefit for individuals with this condition (Collins *et al.*, 1996). However, the issues of context and extrapolation remain difficult, particularly for individuals in primary care. In this domain, some authors take a fairly robust stance. For example, Barbara Starfield (2001) reported that: 'Evidence-based medicine is surely a desirable approach to ensuring the quality of practice; however, existing evidence is not for the most part appropriate for primary care.' Starfield identifies three major flaws in the design of the trials that contribute to the evidence base of primary care. In general, they are seriously underpowered to detect any but the commonest adverse events. This means that when we extrapolate from small or even modest trial populations to large national or even continental populations, we do not know quite what degree of harm we might inflict on those populations. Secondly, they fail to take into account the nature of the primary healthcare that the study subjects receive while they are participating in trials. Starfield herself has shown how the absence or presence of a relationship with a source of primary care can itself be expected to influence the outcome of medical interventions. However, the greatest flaw in the evidence base is the absence of evidence with regard to comorbidity. A defining feature of the randomised controlled trial is that it excludes people with coexisting medical conditions, as this would confound the relationship between intervention and outcome. Yet we know that a quarter of people over the age of 65 years will have three or more comorbid conditions. What we know less about is how the parallel medications for such comorbid conditions might interact over the decades of treatment that such patients will endure.

The issue of concern, then, is the epistemological framework that is deployed to address the genuine uncertainty about treatment benefits in important clinical conditions. However, the type of knowledge that is produced in randomised clinical trials can only provide clarification at the level of populations. We can say what the general direction of advantage is and what the general proportion of risk might be, but even when the evidence is clear (according to the conventions of that model), practitioners are left uneasy about the numbers needed to treat. Consider the evidence with regard to anticoagulation. If we treat 1000 patients, we will prevent between 15 and 40 ischaemic strokes or systemic embolisms, at a cost of inducing between four and six serious haemorrhagic events. Smeeth *et al.* (1999) have drawn attention to the subtle difficulty involved in calculating the numbers needed to treat (NNT) from meta-analyses. Describing them as 'some-times informative, usually misleading', those authors remind us that the numbers needed to treat are sensitive to factors that change the baseline risk, such as outcomes considered, patient characteristics, secular trends in incidence and case fatality, and clinical setting. Pooling the numbers needed to treat derived from meta-analyses may be misleading because the baseline risk often varies between trials. In some ways this is like a social contract with the population at risk – people voluntarily agree to expose themselves to a degree of personal risk in order to benefit both themselves and, by extrapolation, the social whole.

Although clinical decisions in this context are reasonably clear (to clinicians at any rate) in terms of a risk–benefit ratio, this type of approach becomes much more problematic when the clinical intervention itself is set to trigger not following a particular clinical event (such as the confirmation of atrial fibrilla-tion), but at a biochemically determined level of risk. Consider how this population approach now plays out in the field of cardiovascular prevention. If you take just one European guideline for cardiovascular disease, and extract just two risk factors (blood pressure and cholesterol level), three-quarters of the entire European adult population will be identified as being at risk (90% of those over 50 years of age), all requiring external monitoring, and many requiring medica-tion to modify these risk factors. Although nearly all of the risk scores for cardiovascular disease are based on the Framingham risk equation, Fahey and Schroder (2004) have pointed out that this equation does not provide a truly accurate assessment of an individual's cardiovascular risk. Their review suggests that the Framingham figures overestimate both fatal and non-fatal coronary heart disease by about 60%. There is also a documented variation in the way in which these figures are applied, with overestimation occurring in areas where the mortality rate from heart disease is lowest – in England, where the average overestimation is 70%. The overestimation is lowest in areas where the mortality rate from heart disease is highest – in Scotland, where the average overestimate is around 30%.

One discerns in this trend towards clinical intervention at a biochemically determined level of risk a consolidation of the hegemony of the contemporary explanatory model in medicine. There is an authority percolating the provision of clinical advice based on the types of algorithms critiqued by Fahey and Schroder (2004) – reflected, for example, in the precision of the risk calculation figures. The concern here is that patients, on receiving information about their level of risk, might feel bullied into accepting the need for continuous vigilance with regard to their health, medical supervision, and often the consumption of medicines for decades. The philosopher Lionel Trilling cautions us about transactions of this nature: 'Any proposition delivered without a hint of doubt about its validity is a form of bullying' (Delblanco, 2001).

At its most simplistic, it may be unwise to assume that what is statistically significant to the researcher and clinically significant to the doctor will also be personally significant to the patient. Consider the rationale for treating hypertension in a middle-aged man. One could explain to such a patient that 170 middle-aged men would have to have their blood pressure treated for five years in order to prevent one stroke. The patient may well elect to take his chances with the other 169 rather than accept the sick role of a patient who requires daily medication for the rest of his life.

We know that people's attitudes to health are not necessarily or exclusively logical (Johnson, 1995). A patient's attitude to health, and the actions that are taken on that basis, are determined by how that person perceives a particular threat to health, the strength of their belief in the advantages of changing their behaviour to accommodate that threat, and how difficult they believe that behavioural change will be. The beliefs that form attitudes to health are influenced by personal, family, social and demographic factors (Becker, 1974). An individual's actions based on these personal health beliefs are not always apparently rational (Johnson, 1995). For example, research has demonstrated a correlation between the frequency of prescribing psychotropic drugs for mothers and the frequency of prescribing antibiotics for their children in order to treat respiratory infections (Howie and Bigg, 1980). People's actions are influenced by what they think others might expect them to do and by how much importance they attach to those expectations (Fishbein and Azjen, 1975).

This analysis begins to call into question the broader nature of 'significance'. Let us explore this a little further by considering one further criticism of EBM.

Measuring the measurable

The descriptions of EBM and the illustrations of its application, to which I have referred above, were criticised by Ellis *et al.* (1995), among others, for posing only questions the answers to which could be measured, and therefore for implying that if something cannot be measured it is of little value. Rudebeck (1992) expresses it bluntly: 'the requirements of medical research are limited by insisting that an answer should be numeric, otherwise it is not a real answer.' Patients or their representatives pose different types of questions, some of which have numerical answers whereas others are more reflective, philosophical or existential (Dixon and Sweeney, 2000). The problem of the nature of research questions is touched upon in a trenchant critique of academic research in clinical medicine (Rudebeck, 1992). It is worthwhile considering the basis of these criticisms, as they shed light on the epistemologies that compete for focus and meaning in consultations.

Consider the following example, which is taken from one of the articles in the users' guide series published in the *Journal of the American Medical Association* by the EBM Working Group (Laupacis *et al.*, 1994).

Mrs J is a 76-year-old retired schoolteacher who consults because she thinks she is becoming forgetful. The doctor's assessment includes a formal test of her mental state and a series of biochemical tests, the results of which are all normal; this confirms that the patient is suffering from dementia. Her son asks to see the doctor about the problem.

The authors of this article suggest the type of questions which the son might ask the doctor in this situation – questions which can be appropriately dealt with by EBM. They explore two questions: 'What is my mother's prognosis?' and 'Will my mother be alive in five years' time?' They then go on to show how a rigorous appraisal of the relevant literature can produce quantifiable answers to these two questions. The selection of these questions is instructive because they can be given answers that are expressed numerically.

However, consider the example of the 76-year-old woman with dementia. The patient's son may ask the general practitioner the following questions: 'Can my mother be cured?', 'Will she die?' and 'Can her suffering be relieved?' The answers to these questions will certainly involve harnessing skills that are set out usefully by the EBM Working Group. However, the son may also ask 'Why has this happened to her?' and 'What will happen to us now?' He may well reflect on the impact that his mother's illness will have on his own family: 'Should my mother come and stay with us?' and 'What will be the effect on my marriage if she does?'

So it is not always possible to formulate from the patient's presenting story a question whose answer can be obtained from the findings of biomedical research. This should not be interpreted as an inherent weakness of EBM, but it does define its epistemological boundaries.

From the viewpoint of general practice, the concern is that an overemphasis on the questions that can be answered by EBM may run the risk of devaluing those questions that cannot be so expressed – and in turn deflecting attention towards the type of knowledge that populates those questions. The consultation in general practice is not simply a place where a patient seeks scientific answers to questions. Toon (1994) states that: 'The consultation is the patient's forum for coming to understand her illness, not merely a rational understanding, but an under-standing which involves the emotions and which contributes to the growth of the individual.' In a patient-centred consultation, the doctor recognises this and tries to see the illness through the patient's eyes (Peppiatt, 1992). Patients' questions are answered partly by reference to science, but also by reference to what Heath (1995) calls 'the search for meaning.' There is something in all of these descriptions that calls us to consider the relationship of the frameworks from which quantitative and qualitative knowledge arises. They also demand that we revisit the notion of 'significance', which in the conventional biomedical model is presented on two levels – statistical and clinical. I shall pursue this point later in this chapter. First, in order to develop a clearer idea of what a complementary epistemological framework might look like, let us reflect briefly on the broad nature of general practice.

The nature of general practice

Any experience that an individual perceives as threatening or problematic and introduces to the consultation becomes the legitimate concern of the general practitioner. Being competent to deal with the range of potential problems that are encountered in general practice requires a portfolio of intellectual, professional and personal skills. Some aspects of the general practitioner's competence have been described as doctor centred (Guilbert, 1987). They include curative and rehabilitative care, promotion of health, and organisation of preventive activities. Personal skills are equally important components of competence. They are the more patient-centred qualities of competence, and include moral and personal attributes.

In the USA, the American Board of Internal Medicine (1985) stated that: 'A major responsibility of training residents in internal medicine is to stress the importance of the humanistic qualities in the relationship between the patient and physician.' In the UK, these competencies now form a central plank of the recertification processes in the NHS, and it is recommended that 'the recertification of all clinicians should include an assessment of honesty, self-awareness in the professional context, empathy, respect for patient autonomy and confidentiality' (Southgate and Jolly, 1994). The recent acceptance of the new general medical services contract by the medical profession makes the consultation process with patients mandatory, and rewards practices who can show that they have acted upon such consultation (British Medical Association, 2003).

What these initiatives emphasise is the importance of forming a human relationship between the patient and the doctor. The formation of such a relationship is the basis of good consulting, and it requires the ability to identify imaginatively with what a patient experiences subjectively during an illness, and to recognise the validity and importance of that experience for the patient. The term 'human relationship' is used here with a specific meaning to distinguish it from the term 'personal relationship.'

For doctors this distinction is important. In a *personal relationship*, two human beings decide spontaneously to exchange benign sentiments based on mutual care, concern and affection. As the relationship develops, the mutuality and reciprocity become more profound on both sides, and the way in which a personal relationship develops depends on the equal participation of both parties. In a *human relationship*, one person, responding to the human condition of another, seeks to initiate an exchange of benign sentiments (Sweeney, 1992). Human relationships require a genuine concern from the instigator and a positive response from the participant. Such relationships are based on self-knowledge, tolerance, self-confidence, patience and the ability to listen and communicate.

In human relationships the depth of feelings and personal involvement should never be as profound as in a personal relationship, and doctors have a duty to maintain these relationships at an appropriate level. It is this element of control – maintaining the relationship at the appropriate level – which epitomises the difference between the two types of relationship. To illustrate how the tasks of applying best evidence and forming human relationships can be combined, consider the following example.

> *Bert, a former professional soldier, is 63 years old. He consults one day saying that he feels low. The doctor carries out a standard depression inventory to confirm the diagnosis based on Bert's symptoms, and he identifies Bert as a 'case' of depression. Calling on the evidence from clinical trials, he prescribes a tricyclic antidepressant.*

Here the appropriate use of EBM helps the doctor to arrive at the diagnosis of 'depression' by using a validated instrument, and helps the patient to benefit from the best treatment suggested by the relevant clinical trials. After talking further with Bert, the doctor establishes that the depression was initiated by the failure of Bert's son to get into the army. Bert had been a soldier himself, loved the army, and had always wanted his son to join the same regiment. His son also wanted this, but when he failed to do so he became antisocial, drinking too much and experimenting with soft drugs. Bert had found the experience devastating.

This example illustrates the three levels at which a doctor can understand and empathise with a patient. At the first level, the doctor categorises the patient on the basis of established, recognisable patterns of disease – Bert is a 'case' of depression. At the second level, the doctor makes use of the patient's life history to try to understand what has been happening to him – Bert's aspirations for his son are based on his own experiences as a soldier. At the third level, the doctor recognises the uniqueness of the patient's human condition and the *significance* and gravity of the illness from the patient's perspective. Accordingly, in this consultation the use of EBM and the formation of the human relationship are both necessary ingredients of a productive consultation. Neither the diagnostic technique nor the relationship-building skills are in themselves sufficient to constitute an effective consultation. Heath (1995) identifies two fundamental roles for the general practitioner, namely acting as an interpreter and guardian at the interface between illness and disease, and acting as a witness to the patient's experience of both.

Consider the patient with end-stage chronic obstructive airways disease, for whom no more can be done by the respiratory specialists. Such patients may linger on in a terminal state for months or years, deriving gradually less benefit from steroids, antibiotics and bronchodilators. Their burden of illness and the burden on their carers need to be witnessed and supported despite the failure of biomedicine to help them.

The distinction which appears to be fundamental for the general practitioner is that between illness and disease. Illness may exist without disease, which is a narrower reconfiguration of the patient's story based on biomedical science (Kleinman, 1988). Doctors have a duty to explore the meaning of illness, recognising its potential origin in unhappiness, unfavourable socio-economic circumstances or chronically unsatisfactory personal relationships (Morris, 1998). They need to recognise that the severity of an illness can be a function of an individual's health beliefs and particular life circumstances (Becker, 1974). There is a further duty to protect patients from overenthusiastic interpretation of illness as disease. Kleinman (1988) cautions doctors against the 'over-literal interpretation of accounts best understood metaphorically.' Here the doctor works with the patient to make sense of the patient's experience in the context of the rest of the patient's life. This has been described elsewhere as the hermeneutic (Toon, 1994) or biographical (Marinker, 1994) tasks of the doctor.

What this analysis emphasises is the gravitas and relevance of knowledge that arises out of context, out of personal narrative and, crucially, out of the interaction between doctor and patient in consultations. This interaction – the undisputed basis of any relationship – is a mutually changing process, as it gradually and subtly changes both participants, their own relationship, and the way in which they interact with others.

The EBM Working Group argued that many patients are being denied the benefits of evidence from well-conducted clinical trials (Sackett and Rosenberg, 1995). The evidence supports this view (Haines and Jones, 1994). Accordingly, doctors have a responsibility to acquire new skills in accessing, evaluating and applying the results of the vast number of clinical studies that are now being published worldwide. In pursuit of this end, the integration of EBM into the clinical work of general practice is both necessary and timely. The danger lies in regarding EBM as the only and last word in the pursuit of clinical quality and the search for relevant evidence. For example, the conventional approach to the task of modifying the behaviour of doctors has been to offer educational inputs or to formulate clinical guidelines. To some extent these work (Grimshaw and Russell, 1993). However, the decision to change a clinical habit can be the result of a series of influences, which may not be dealt with by a conventional approach where the researcher has to guess in advance which intervention is most likely to succeed. Yet patients, or their representatives, also pose different types of questions, some of which have numerical answers, while others have answers that are more reflective, philosophical or existential (Dixon and Sweeney, 2000). The problem of the nature of research questions is touched upon in a trenchant critique of academic research in clinical medicine, which argues that the requirements of medical research are limited by insisting 'that an answer should be numeric, otherwise it is not a real answer' (Rudebeck, 1992).

However, this is not a dichotomous taxonomy of questions, numerical or otherwise. Mary Midgley (1992) states that: 'The mere presence of an emotional factor in any kind of decision does not take it out of the realm of rational thought. All our thinking involves emotional factors as well as rational ones, just as every physical object has size as well as shape. These are not alternatives. The presence of one does not mean the absence of another.' The challenge lies in integrating one with the other. Midgley (1992) expresses it thus: 'We need ways of thinking which are unifying enough to give us guiding patterns, but not so strongly reductive as to leave out something important.'

A seminal study of doctors' reasons for changing their prescribing behaviour illustrates this point (Armstrong et al., 1996). The researchers encouraged the clinicians to explain and understand their own reasons for altering their pre-scribing habits. The researchers identified three models of change. Some doctors altered their prescribing policy as a result of the sheer pressure to move in a certain direction, evidence for which came in various forms, such as articles, letters from consultants, and talks that they had attended. A second model of change was more abrupt, and occurred in response to near 'clinical disasters' or to changes in prescribing initiated by a second doctor, sometimes a locum. A third group of doctors seemed to embrace change in general more enthusiastically. They were more prepared to be influenced by a variety of sources, some of which would be regarded as conventionally authoritative, such as journal articles, while others would not, such as magazine advertisements and television programmes.

This important article is saying something fundamental about personal epistemologies – that is, the type of knowledge that an individual regards as 'true' or valuable. One can have what psychologists call a 'naive' epistemology where, at risk of simplifying a complex literature, knowledge is regarded as something certain, carefully teased out of issues that are seen as solvable puzzles. Conventionally, people who hold such naive epistemologies defer to experts and authorities as the source of valuable knowledge. At the other end of a knowledge continuum, one can hold a more complex view of the nature of knowledge, seeing it as always contingent, uncertain and arising from a range of domains, including personal narrative and context as well as more objective 'factual' knowledge. Here individuals tend to be more anti-condescensionist, regarding authority as always potentially fallible. At its extreme, this stance may be described as postmodern, sceptical and constructionist. It can, for example, be seen in the lack of authority of secularism and science in contemporary society in the USA (Pederson, 2005). One is driven, through this analysis, to consider *how* we know things, to entertain the possibility that there is more than one way of knowing and that, by implication, the current explanatory model in medicine, predicated as it is on biomedical positivism, is one way of knowing, which reflects a particular world-view and a preference for a particular type of knowledge. At the spearhead of medicine's explanatory model we find the notion of significance – the convention whereby we judge whether knowledge produced through this framework's processes is worthy of interest or action. If we now consider that there may be more than one way of knowing, then we should revisit the notion of significance, take a view of its limitations, and theorise about how it might usefully be extended. This brings us to the notion of personal significance (Sweeney *et al.*, 1998).

Personal significance

At stake in this part of the argument are the nature, importance and relevance of subjectivity, a notion of little relevance within the conventional medical model. In that context, subjective evidence is anathema. In this context, EBM is almost always doctor centred. It focuses on the doctor's objective interpretation of the evidence, and it either jeopardises or diminishes the importance of human relationships and the role of the other partner in the consultation – the patient.

Earlier in the chapter I described the current position, whereby the importance of research evidence is weighted with mathematical models which, within each study, describe its importance according to two levels of significance – statistical and clinical. There is no mystery attached to statistical significance – it is simply the mathematical likelihood that the result did not occur by chance. Clinical significance, we agreed, describes what the results would mean if applied to a population similar to that studied. But therein lay its limitation. Although clinical significance attempts to clarify the potential impact of the research, it only applies to populations or groups of patients. As clinicians, particularly in primary care, we still face the difficulty of extrapolating such population-derived information to the individual patient, who may not enter the consulting room with a discrete one-dimensional problem that can readily be turned into an answerable question (Charlton, 1995b; *Lancet*, 1995; Greenhalgh, 1996).

In a traditional model, new research findings are passed to the professional community via the conventional pathways of peer-reviewed journals and clinical meetings. The next step involves the receipt of that evidence by the wider health community – the move from Rogers' (1983) earlier adopters to the majority and ultimately the so-called 'laggards.' Evidence from medical research reaches doctors and patients in different ways, but it is self-evident that doctors do not always hear of new research findings first. Increasingly, such findings are rapidly disseminated through the media, or are learned about through family or friends. And patients are not passive recipients of information – they have their own ways of interpreting and responding to new findings. The crucial step in dissemination of clinical information occurs during the interaction between doctor and patient, when an individual practitioner interprets and explains the clinical information for and with an individual patient during a one-to-one consultation. This is not a simple transaction. The term 'personal significance' helps us to understand the components of this part of the consultation from the perspective both of the clinician and of the person (patient) who may benefit from the information. Although it is acknowledged that factors associated with the doctor can affect the way in which a message is transmitted and interpreted, what really matters is what the message means to the patient (Balint, 1957).

Once again, in this critique of statistical and clinical significance I do not intend to diminish their vital contribution to clinical thinking. The crucial advantage that these mathematical models constantly seek is the reproducibility of the data produced by investigation. My aim, rather, is to debate their limitations, and in so doing to call into question their intellectual impregnability.

Consider first the derivation of statistical significance. The accepted value for statistical significance, $P < 0.05$, is based on the understanding that in any Gaussian distribution of a continuous variable, 95% of the data are included in a zone that is covered by 1.96 standard deviations of the mean. The 5% of data that do not fall within this span should be regarded as inconsistent with the main distribution. Statistical significance is the term used to indicate the probability of clinical data falling within this span (Feinstein, 1992). Is this valuable? Indeed it is, but let us think of the notion in the context of clinical care.

The primary reasoning behind this calculation of P does not fit easily with the distribution of many kinds of data that are found in clinical medicine. In addition, this type of frequentist theory, which has dominated medical research for much of the last century, creates a dichotomy in which results are regarded as either significant or not. Arguing in favour of a change of model towards Bayesian statistics, Lilford and Braunholtz (1996) proposed that dichotomous results ('either it is or it isn't') do not take into account relevant evidence obtained outside the index experiment, which may be important in formulating clinical policies. Out of such dichotomous reasoning emerges the paradox that very small differences will eventually 'become' significant if repeated often enough in a very large series. Thirdly, human factors can also affect statistical interpretation. As we discussed earlier in the chapter, a single summary out-come statistic cannot capture satisfactorily the heterogeneity of the combined experience of the individuals in a clinical trial. Such calculations fail to address the issue of auxometry (the rate of progression of illness). Patients who have the same disease at the point of entry in a trial may have different patterns of the illness, with different rates of progression and clinical features, which can affect both treatment and prognosis (Feinstein, 1992). Thus the importance of statistical significance lies in the early stages of the interpretation of research findings.

Although the results of a clinical trial may be *statistically* significant, the clinician is helped to interpret such evidence with the calculations that collectively constitute *clinical* significance. In general there are four key calculations, namely absolute risk reduction, risk ratio, relative risk reduction (the complement of risk ratio expressed as a percentage) and the concept of the number needed to treat (the inverse of the absolute risk reduction) (Sackett *et al.*, 1985).

These concepts, particularly the number needed to treat, have been of especial value to clinicians in helping them to interpret the results of trials. However, what remains unresolved is the precise boundary at which a distinction between two means or two rates can be regarded as quantitatively significant – to the same extent that the stochastic component of statistical significance lies at 0.05. In their review, Burnand *et al.* (1990) noted the boundaries that were being used by general medical journals to trigger such quantitative decisions in research that contrasts two means, two rates or two correlation coefficients. They found that this boundary was reached when the ratio of the smaller to the larger mean was greater than 1.2, where the odds ratio was greater than 2.2, and where the r-value for the correlation coefficient was greater than 0.32. However, these conclusions are based only on the authors' reporting of the interpretative comments of the component studies in the review – they do not represent a consensus view.

Clinical significance is thus an important additional factor that can aid the interpretation of research findings for regional, district or practice populations. However, the whole aim of producing such evidence and calculating statistics is to clarify the clinical dilemma for the patient. Thus the most important application of such findings lies in the context of the individual consultation, during which such information is tailored to the individual personal context of the patient.

Personal significance adds a further dimension, and is the key to the transfer of an idea to, and the evaluation and interpretation of that idea by, the doctor and the patient together. Personal significance is thus a dialectic consisting of a contribution from the practitioner, who outlines the concept as he or she understands it, and the person who receives and evaluates the new idea. At the heart of this definition is the interaction between the two participants in a consultation – and it is this that drives the definition towards a greater appreciation of subjectivity (and indeed inter-subjectivity, the process of their inter-action). In the context of the argument that is unfolding in this book, we are close to considering – if we accept the processes involved in personal significance – a new way of knowing.

The contribution of the doctor is threefold, namely evaluating the research evidence, exploring the patient's philosophy of health, and delivering an opinion that is based on a synthesis of the two. Doctors evaluate evidence in different ways. Usually they will have an opportunity to evaluate information independently, before engaging in a consultation. But doctors are people, too – they are not immune from fears, prejudices and attitudes to health by virtue of having received a medical education. The evaluation process is not simply an intellectual procedure, but includes both cognitive and intuitive components. This process has been best described by Neighbour (1987) as an 'inner consultation' in which a dialogue takes place between what he terms the organiser (the logical part of the process) and the responder (the more intuitive component).

Doctors conduct an inner consultation with biomedical evidence before deciding how to apply it. Although the doctor's organiser responds in an analytical, logical way, the evaluation of new evidence is also influenced by the doctor's background, experience and other individual factors. Thus the doctor's responder will act in a more intuitive manner, using pattern recognition and the association of ideas in a Gestalt manner. The responder is sensitive to internal messages determined by the doctor's feelings and emotion, and this affects the interpretation of information in a way that recognises context, experience, apprehensions, failures and successes. This elevates and dignifies the doctor's subjectivity.

Furthermore, the consultation occurs at one point in what may be a long-standing doctor–patient relationship. Such relationships are dynamic and ever changing, so that the interaction between organiser and responder, and between the product of that dialogue and the influence of the patient, evolves over time. For the experienced doctor the logical (organising) processes become less important, and are replaced by historical pattern analysis or script recognition from exposure to previous similar problems – a responder function. This is what distinguishes the thinking of novices from that of experts (Van der Vleuten and Newble, 1995), and focuses the analysis on the interaction between doctor and patient.

The second part of the doctor's role in personal significance involves exploring the patient's health philosophy. The clinician and patient may have different priorities, so the traditional healthcare philosophy of the medical profession may not be shared by an individual person. For the most part, medicine assumes that disease-free longevity is desirable, even at the expense of matters that patients consider to be of more immediate and substantial concern (Landau and Gustaffson, 1984). Let us recall the case of Mrs B. She was conveying a despair and hopelessness about her predicament, to the effect that, put bluntly, she no longer wanted to live. Consequently, she began to take decisions about the care of her diabetes that were incompatible with expert professional advice. Mrs B is telling us something extremely important. If patients' priorities differ from those of the clinician, the quality of medical evidence matters little, as the clinician's advice based upon it will be ignored.

Finally, the style and method of communication may also affect the message, and contribute to the patient's personal significance. A doctor's own experience, either privately or professionally, will influence the words and nuances that he or she uses in discussion. For example, the doctor who wrongly diagnosed a benign breast cyst that turned out to be a breast carcinoma will alter his future behaviour and management of women who present with fibroadenosis in a way that is coloured by this experience. It is almost impossible for doctors to be clinically dispassionate or completely neutral about a topic – their view is a product of both cognitive and experiential evidence. This aspect of the definition of personal significance encourages us even further to focus on the interaction between the two participants in the consultation. The crucial point here is that this interaction is unpredictable – its outcome is emergent, in the sense that it cannot be known in advance. And it is serendipitous, constantly at the whim of the frailty of the human predicament. We shall revisit these features of personal significance in

Chapter 5, when I discuss the complexity theorist Ralph Stacey's definition of complex responsive processes (Stacey, 2000).

However, it is the patient's contribution that is more important in creating personal significance. In a consultation the patient adds to previous intellectual and emotional understanding of an illness experience (Heath, 1995; Cromarty, 1996). Patients are not passive recipients waiting for doctors to make decisions about their health. The evidence suggests that the more actively patients participate in consultations, the better controlled are their chronic diseases (Kaplan *et al.*, 1989). Attitudes to health are not exclusively logical. People's attitudes to health, and the decisions that they take, are determined by how they perceive a particular threat to health, their belief in the advantages to be gained from a change in behaviour to accommodate that threat, and how difficult they believe that behaviour change to be. The beliefs that form attitudes to health are influenced by personal and family factors, and also by social and demographic factors (Becker, 1974). Actions that are based upon these beliefs are not always rational – they can be emotional or habitual (Johnson, 1995). The actions that patients take are influenced by what they think others might expect them to do, and by how much importance they attach to those expectations (Fishbein and Azjen, 1975). Of course this analysis applies equally to the doctor as a person, not just as a professional. As Kant said, 'we see things not as they are, but as we are' (Russell, 1961). This firmly roots the definition of personal significance in the patient's personal history, personal narrative and personal epistemology. The subjectivity of the interaction has become the major feature of the definition.

Summary

The contemporary explanatory model in medicine boasts a long and illustrious pedigree, which was outlined in the previous chapter. From that tradition has emerged the model of EBM, which has contributed directly and extensively to improvements in patient care, and which has anchored critical appraisal of evidence firmly in the clinical arena. In this chapter we have reflected generically on the criticisms of the model. By considering the individual criticisms, we have been encouraged to interrogate the nature of diagnosis in clinical practice, the properties of a randomised controlled trial, the type of knowledge produced by that process, and the conventions (statistical and clinical significance) whereby a value can be attached to such knowledge. I argue that this process has helped to define the limitations of these two conventional levels of significance, and encouraged, by way of a response, the introduction of a third level of significance. At stake in the definition of that third level – personal significance – is the centrality of subjectivity and interaction, and of emergence and serendipity, in the clinical encounter. We are forced to consider that this represents a different 'way of knowing.' It is now appropriate to explore the intellectual pedigree of this 'way of knowing', by tracing the historical antecedents of a constructivist, naturalistic way of understanding the world. Although these terms might be unfamiliar to the jobbing clinician (and indeed to your humble author), they might be more easily recognised as the building blocks for the principles of qualitative research. This subject is explored in the next chapter.

Chapter 4

The naturalistic tradition: historical overview of the epistemological origins of qualitative research

Introduction

This chapter describes the evolution of a second intellectual tradition, described as naturalistic. This tradition is characterised by a search for truth predicated on scepticism, a constant comparison of the natural and the social world, and the emergence of a socially constructed ontology. The evolution of the naturalistic tradition has led to the development of sociology as a legitimate domain of enquiry, and of qualitative research methods as appropriate tools for exploring the meaning of human actions. The history of thinking from the seventeenth century to the present day illustrates how philosophers' struggle with the notion of 'truth' has influenced the development of these qualitative research methods.

The purpose of this chapter is to encourage us to compare this naturalistic tradition with the development of the scientific tradition set out in the previous chapter, and to prepare us to consider a third intellectual tradition, predicated on non-linearity, which we shall explore in the next chapter. The key idea to bear in mind is the relationship between the way we explain things, the type of knowledge we consequently prefer to create in order to furnish those explanations, and a fundamental world-view which underpins that way of thinking. Putting those thoughts in more philosophical language, I argue that these three traditions (scientific, naturalistic and non-linear) are predicated on different but complementary ontologies. Their comparison reveals how each has created its own epistemological framework with which to populate that world-view in the form of an explanatory model.

Historical development of qualitative research methods

It is convenient, following the proposals of Auguste Comte (1798–1857) in his *Course of Positive Philosophy* (Comte, 1875), to consider the history of a naturalistic tradition in three periods.

- The first era covers roughly the seventeenth to the nineteenth centuries. During this period the natural and social sciences were indistinguishable, and every form of scientific enquiry was regarded as philosophical (Dunn *et al.*, 1992). This period includes the work of Montaigne and Bacon, sets out the basis of Cartesian duality and doubt, and includes the contributions of Berkeley and Hume.

- The second period includes the writing of Kant, Comte, Weber and Mill. During this period positivism was developed, and the hierarchy of the sciences was described, placing the physical sciences at the pinnacle of knowledge.
- The third period covers the twentieth century. Tensions between qualitative and quantitative approaches arose and then matured from a position of opposition to one of greater collaboration (Rossman, 1985).

The first period: the seventeenth century – a point of departure

The seventeenth century, regarded by some as the beginning of the modern world, can be taken as a convenient starting point for this historical overview of qualitative research (Grbich, 1999). At this time, the dominant intellectual authority lay with the Roman Catholic Church. Although the Church approved scholarship, it only afforded seniority and influence to scholars who did not challenge its authority. As Hawthorn (1976) points out, it resisted any rise in a rational form of human enquiry – this was really a political dislike of challenge to its static epistemological position of an unchanged and unchanging Creation. The church's assertion of the privileged position accorded to divine final cause would have been fatally weakened by the rise of a science that revealed 'divine' purpose in what we would now describe as a naturalistic way. The notion of absolute truth dominated (Crosby, 1997), and was strategically linked to the concept of power. However, the Roman Catholic Church could not stifle the frustration caused by its inflexible position, nor could it eliminate the inexorable rise in scepticism that characterised subsequent Renaissance science. And it is with Renaissance science that a more detailed description of the history of qualitative research can begin (Murphy *et al.*, 1998). The names of the main contributors during this period, and their principal contributions in the context of this chapter, are presented in Table 4.1. Although this may be an egregious conflation of their contribution to human knowledge, its purpose is to clarify their relevance to the propositions explored in this book.

Table 4.1 Key figures during the first period

Philosopher	Dates	Principal contribution in the context of this chapter
Montaigne	1533–1592	Development of sceptical approach to knowledge
Francis Bacon	1561–1626	The notion of induction, permitting generalities to be accumulated from particular observations. Embryo of the scientific method
Thomas Hobbes	1588–1679	Hyperbolic doubt. How do we know how accurate our observations are? Embryo of social construction
René Descartes	1596–1650	Cartesian duality and Cartesian doubt. Application of mechanical and mathematical principles to natural phenomena
George Berkeley	1685–1735	Immaterialism and further origins of socially constructed ideas of knowledge
David Hume	1711–1776	The nature of uncertain knowledge, our knowledge of the future, and of causality
Adam Smith	1723–1790	The integration of the natural and social sciences (or natural and moral philosophy). Combination of research methods in the *Wealth of Nations*

The Renaissance and the Reformation

An increase in scepticism characterised intellectual progress during the Renaissance and Reformation, and is epitomised by the work of Montaigne (1533–1592) and Bacon (1561–1626). Bacon exhorted scientists to undertake a completely 'fresh' examination of particulars in an orderly and considered manner. 'There remains simple experience which, if taken as it comes, is called accident', he wrote. 'But if sought for experiment, the true method commences with experience truly ordered and digested' (Bacon, 1858). Montaigne, on the other hand, was more explicitly sceptical. *'Que sais-je?'* was his personal motto (Burke, 1981).

The notion of experimentation was much broader at this time, and could refer to any occasion during which one tested out the validity of a proposition – this could include what we would regard as natural experiments in contemporary qualitative research (Murphy *et al.*, 1998). Bacon advocated induction. He suggested that one could draw up particularities of observation from experience and experiments, and combine them to create lesser, then greater generalities (Tuck, 1993). Although Bacon illustrated his methods mostly by reference to physical phenomena, he advocated that a sceptical approach should also be taken to the study of history, literature and philosophy. The historian Lester King (1982) asserts that it is in Bacon that we find the principal elements of the modern scientific method, as he recognised the need for controls, verification and reduction of bias (Greaves, 1996).

Hyperbolic doubt, Cartesian doubt and duality

The philosophers who followed Bacon, notably Hobbes (1588–1679), who was in fact a younger contemporary, developed scepticism in a much more fundamental way, focusing on the very act of observation itself. The radical nature of their scepticism came to be known as hyperbolic doubt (Tuck, 1993).

The central core of hyperbolic doubt concerns the nature of observation. How can we know that our observations are accurate reflections of the external world? These questions arose in the seventeenth century mainly as a result of developments in optics, which at that time strayed into areas which we would probably now regard as the domain of psychology, and Hobbes himself was much inspired by Galileo (Russell, 1961). Seventeenth-century advances in optics encouraged scientists to define more precisely and at the same time to doubt the veracity of perceptions. Indeed the use of mirrors and lenses was sometimes associated with intrigue and falsehood (Hurwitz B, personal communication). Although these advances might allow individuals to make observations that would be impossible with the naked eye, that same eye could easily be tricked by their misuse. So how could accurate and critical observations be distinguished from unreliable ones?

Philosophers in the seventeenth century regarded this issue as a practical problem rather than an ontological one. They proposed, as a way of closing the logical gap between sensory observation and interpretation, that observations should be regarded as *signs* of the world. In doing so, they still relied on divine inspiration, arguing that God would not play tricks on his creatures, and that at the very least a thinking body could be certain of its own existence and the correctness of immediate sensations. In the end we could trust our perceptions, they argued.

This is encapsulated in the well-known dictum, *cogito ergo sum*, of Descartes (1596–1650). Descartes epitomised the scepticism which flourished at that time in his explication of Cartesian doubt (Russell, 1961). The irreducibility of the 'I' led Descartes to assert that the soul (mind) was different from the body – this Cartesian duality would influence medical thinking for the next 200 years. Descartes' influence on the subsequent development of epistemologies is central. His notion of truth was predicated on a view of the world as linked to but separate from subjective interpretations, emotions, reflection and consciousness (Descartes, 1912). The reality constructed from such truths was measurable and controllable – by using logic and mathematics one could make accurate predictions of future events (Crosby, 1997). In this lies the kernel of the scientific method and subsequent positivist epistemology.

On the other hand, the importance of hyperbolic doubt was that it created a rather different notion of how scientific enquiry should proceed. Rather than seeing and understanding the world by inferring the rules that may govern it, science began to regard the world as the creation of our observations, rather than regarding our observations as being a copy of it. Our own observations and interpretations, then, could be a proper focus for enquiry – and for some, the origins of social construction.

The approach developed by Hobbes and others arose from their concern about Bacon's reliance on induction (Murphy *et al.*, 1998). Induction is the process of proceeding from a list of singular statements to a universal statement. It is defined by Chalmers (1982) as follows: 'If a large number of A's have been observed under a variety of conditions, and if all those observed A's without exception possessed the property B, then all A's have the property B.' Dilman (1973) describes induction as occurring 'where we reason from a piece of information, however complex or elaborate this may be, to a conclusion which is logically independent of it.' By contrast, he argues, deduction occurs when 'the relation between premise and conclusion, by virtue of which I am justified in inferring the latter from the former, is internal and can be gathered from the premise and conclusion alone. What the conclusion states is already contained in the premise' (Dilman, 1973).

Collingwood (1946) points out that Bacon asserted that one of his contributions was to develop induction as a break from the dominance of deductive reasoning which had characterised most historical writing up until then. It was such deductive reasoning, for example, that allowed medieval history to be viewed as illustrations of the Divine Plan. Such revelations contained useful (divine) knowledge, because its premises determined its conclusions (Collingwood, 1946). However, the sceptics were arguing about the assumptions which underpinned the very particular observations that constituted the cornerstone of the inductive method.

Immaterialism: the origins of social constructionism?

The approach to philosophical enquiry predicated upon profound scepticism was subsequently developed by Bishop George Berkeley (1685–1735), and it is to him that Murphy *et al.* (1998) and Bloor (1976) attribute much of the foundations of contemporary qualitative research. Berkeley is important in philosophy because of his denial of the existence of matter – that is, immaterialism. His principles, which were all set out when he was relatively young, are best seen in his *Dialogues of Hylas and Philonous*, which was written in 1713 (Berkeley, 1967). Hylas, who represents the scientifically educated common-sense person, debates with Philonous (effectively Berkeley himself) about the nature of material substance. 'Can there be anything so repugnant to common sense than not to believe in matter?', asks Hylas. Philonous does not deny the existence of sensible things, but asserts that one does not see the *causes* of colours, or hear the *causes* of sounds. The reality of sensible things consists, he says, of being perceived (Russell, 1961). His philosophy was irreverently captured in the following limerick, and reply, by Monsignor Ronald Knox:

> *There was a young man who said God*
> *Must think it exceedingly odd*
> *If he finds that this tree*
> *Continues to be*
> *When there's no one about in the quad.*

Reply:

> *Dear Sir:*
> *Your astonishment's odd: I am always about in the quad.*
> *And that's why the tree*
> *Will continue to be,*
> *Since observed by,*
> *Yours faithfully,*

> *God.*

(Quoted in Russell, 1961)

It was unnecessary, Berkeley argued, to propose the idea of a separate world composed of physical matter, because what was much more important was the way in which human beings classified and organised the world, and acted according to those classifications. While insisting that he started from a common-sense view of the world, Berkeley recognised a number of objections to his position. First, the most obvious objection was the idea that objects would cease to exist if we did not attend to them – the main message in the limerick quoted above. Secondly, if material objects were irrelevant, then the world as we know it would have the same attributes or lack of attributes as dreams, illusions and fantasies. Finally, there is a seemingly obvious distinction between a real blow and an imagined blow, between the imagining of being struck by a blow and the actual experience of it. Berkeley (1967) responded to these arguments by stating that ideas can be distinguished from each other by their having a different nature or order, such that the ideas of reality are stronger and exhibit some regularity. The quality of ideas also allows us to establish procedures for counting or deciding what is real (Russell, 1961).

Within the context of this chapter, Berkeley's influence on qualitative research lies in this rather arcane notion of immaterialism. From Berkeley's perspective, what we know *is* the way in which we construct the world – there is nothing knowable other than minds and their contents (Berkeley, 1967). This does seem recognisable in the notion of social constructionism upon which much qualitative research rests. Berkeley starts from a common-sense view of the world, resisting the introduction of theoretical assumptions or technical notions. According to

Collingwood (1946), Berkeley was at pains not to demean science by this route. His main point was not to make the mistake of assuming that science offered absolute truths. New scientific hypotheses that were more predictive than their antecedent hypotheses were indeed more powerful, but despite their predictive capacity, they were always vulnerable to alternative descriptions and more accurate results. Many contemporary qualitative researchers, drawing on Berkeley's influence, continue to adhere to the view that it is entirely appropriate to study the world from the perspective of social construction, including a social construction of the world created by science (Chalmers, 1982).

The application of Berkeley's approach in recent research in medicine is illustrated by a paper by Bloor (1976) on decision making among ENT surgeons. Bloor observed 11 ENT surgeons in various clinic settings, gradually drawing together a picture of the various processes and procedures that the surgeons used to decide whether a patient who had been referred should be listed for adenotonsillectomy. He analysed the data inductively, identifying the way in which each surgeon took their clinical histories and made decisions. Both of these activities, history taking and decision making, differed among the 11 specialists. The data suggested that the surgeons attributed different weights to the same physical findings. From Berkeley's perspective, the surgeons were socially constructing their decisions in this context in a way that reflected their experience of the domain.

Causality

Although the main focus of Berkeley's philosophy was on immaterialism, much less prominence was given to the notion of causality, which Berkeley formulated merely as a linkage between two repeatedly observed phenomena. It was David Hume (1711–1776) who refined the notion of causality during the eighteenth century (Russell, 1961). In his *Treatise on Human Nature*, Hume (1739) identified two kinds of statement. Drawing on algebra and geometry, the first statement, which he termed *impressions*, concerned statements that can be shown to be demonstrably true because the conclusions are inherent in the ideas themselves. An example is the proposition from Euclidean geometry that the square of the hypotenuse is equal to the sum of the squares of the opposite two sides. Contained in the section of his treatise entitled *Of Knowledge and Probability*, the second kind of statement from Hume's work related to all knowledge deriving from empirical data that cannot be directly demonstrated. Thus it includes all our knowledge about the future (Hume, 1975). His discussion here has real relevance for current research in medicine and for qualitative and social science research, as it explores the notion of predictability. For Hume, the notion that the sun would *not* rise tomorrow was as logically intelligible as the statement 'The sun will rise tomorrow.' However, we disbelieve one and firmly believe the other. Hume's description of causation had three components, namely contiguity in time and space, priority in time (the cause preceding the effect), and a necessary connection between the two (Hume, 1739). Essentially, Hume was arguing that we observe regular conjunctions, and it is the regularity of these conjunctions that creates the notion of necessity about any connection between a regularly conjoined antecedent and subsequent event. This is falling short of the notion of absolute causation. Hume's answer was to say that although we cannot be sure of the laws of physics, nature continues in such a uniform way that we can treat conjunctions as causal for practical purposes (Hume, 1739).

In the context of contemporary medicine, Hume might ask how we can predict that the effect of a treatment which has worked well in many thousands of previous patients will work well in a particular patient with the same condition. The regularity of the connection between the treatment and subsequent beneficial outcome in the past does not confer any absolute certainty of its benefit in a particular case in the future. For contemporary qualitative research, Hume's legacy also lies in his integration of the natural and social sciences. The first social scientists – Smith and Ferguson in Scotland, and Montesquieu and Vico in France and Italy, respectively – were heavily influenced by Hume's support for induction (Schneider, 1967). One could induce generalisation or regularities about society, Hume argued, only if they were based on extensive observations.

Adam Smith's *An Inquiry into the Nature and Causes of the Wealth of Nations*, first published in 1776, uses a wide range of methods to present its conclusions, including statistics, historical documents, written accounts and personal observations (Smith, 1976, 1993). These two notions, namely Berkeley's immaterialism and Hume's constant conjunction, heavily influenced the way in which qualitative researchers formulated ideas up to and throughout the twentieth century (Murphy *et al.*, 1998).

The second period: positivism and the hierarchy of the sciences

The second period covered in this analysis includes the work of Kant, Comte, Weber and Mill. During this period positivism was developed and the hierarchy of the sciences was described, placing the physical sciences at the pinnacle of knowledge. The names of the main contributors and their principal contributions in the context of this chapter are presented in Table 4.2.

Table 4.2 Key figures in the second period

Philosopher	Dates	Principal contribution in the context of this chapter
Immanuel Kant	1724–1804	Observations were theory driven. Exploration of the balance between experience and systems of thought (phenomenon and noumenon), reflected in the balance between data and theory in contemporary research
Auguste Comte	1798–1857	The introduction of positivism. Presenting the sciences in a hierarchy, with the physical sciences at the pinnacle
John Stuart Mill	1806–1873	Exploring the notion of positivism introduced by the French philosopher Auguste Comte. Embedding the process of induction in the social sciences
Max Weber	1864–1920	Rejection of the notion that quantification and measurement were the only proper tools for a scientific enquiry (the word 'science' meaning rigorous and precise)

Kant and the emergence of social science

Among the issues that philosophers were grappling with at this time was the question of what constitutes reliable knowledge – as important a notion now for contemporary medical research as it was then for Immanuel Kant (1724–1804) and John Stuart Mill (1806–1873), two of the philosophers who were most directly influenced by Hume and Berkeley. Mill in particular explored the theme of how people could grasp reliable knowledge. He developed both the notion of induction and the notion of causal laws. In the context of this chapter, the importance of his contribution lies in applying both of these to the fields of psychology and economics, as well as sociology and history. Perhaps more importantly, the rather difficult writings of Kant developed thinking from where Hume and Berkeley left off. It is important to spend some time considering Kant's main points because of their influence on German and American qualitative social science in the nineteenth and twentieth centuries.

Kant rejected the view that our knowledge of the world is founded simply and exclusively on our experience of it. Although experience provided the contents of knowledge, Kant argued in *Critique of Pure Reason*, reason was also necessary to provide a structure or order. While the outer world causes only the matter of sensation, our own mental faculties order this matter in space and time, and supply the concepts by which we understand experience (Russell, 1961). He distinguished between analytic and synthetic propositions, and between empirical and a priori propositions. An analytic proposition is one in which the predicate is part of the subject – for example, a fat man is a man. A synthetic proposition is one that is not analytic, and so includes everything we can know through experience. An empirical proposition is one that we can know only by sense-perception, either directly or via reliable testimony – for example, the facts of history and geography. An a priori proposition is one that, although elicited by experience, is seen to have a basis other than experience – all the laws of mathematics are in this sense a priori (Russell, 1961).

In this sense, Kant's thinking influenced contemporary commentators on the role of science, fuelling the debate about theory-driven observations, elegantly explored by Chalmers (1982). Kant argued that we cannot usefully and productively focus our gaze on the world unless we have a prior theory which directs our observations. The form of knowledge that derives from such an activity is objective in the sense of being independent of the observer. Kant applied the term 'transcendent idealism' to this idea to suggest its ability to overcome the notion that knowledge is derived purely from (sensory) ideas of the world. Although we draw knowledge from our sensations, Kant argued, we also have knowledge of theories and concepts which organise the way in which we experience these sensations. Scruton (1982), in a commentary on this work, writes: 'A mind without concepts would have no capacity to think; equally, a mind armed with concepts but with no sensory data to which they could be applied would have nothing to think *about*' (his emphasis).

In Kant's work, theory and data are given equal status. Kant ascribed distinguishing terms to these two notions. A *phenomenon* is what appears to us in perception, and it consists of two parts, namely the sensation, and the part due to our subjective apparatus, which allows us to order or classify the perception. *Noumenon*, in Kant's taxonomy, refers more to systems of thought, a mechanism by which ideas can be classified and not something that can be directly experienced (Russell, 1961). Murphy *et al.* (1998) argue that this taxonomy had a major influence on subsequent social theory. By the 1870s, this kind of epistemological debate was influencing the methods and practice of the social scientists (Adorno *et al.*, 1976). In contemporary terms, this debate is expressed in the arguments about whether the social sciences are informed by abstract or empirical knowledge.

Addressing this issue, the German economist Menger identified two types of knowledge, in a classification broadly similar to that of Kant, namely a knowledge of concrete instances and a knowledge of forms or types. Types can be experienced in individual form, which allows us to characterise them. However, it is our understanding of typicality that makes prediction possible. Menger, who was an economist, was able to distinguish between theoretical economics, an analysis of type, and historical economics, concentrating on individual cases.

At the turn of the nineteenth century, debate about this distinction was aided by considering the idea that disciplines could be categorised to reflect the distinction between type and case – between what came to be called nomothetic disciplines (concerned with laws and generalisations) and ideographic disciplines (concerned with specific instances) (Freund, 1968). For example, a nomothetic study of society could be part of a natural science concerned with looking at the regularities in institutions and individuals. An ideographic study of the same society could generate a cultural science, concerning itself with questions about what leads us to think about that society in a particular way. This is an important distinction to bear in mind when reflecting on contemporary research. The kind of evidence that is produced by the randomised trial is in the form of generalisations – more nomothetic than ideographic. This leaves the clinician with the ideographic challenge of applying such nomothetic evidence in individual consultations. The value of considering the taxonomy as complementary, rather than as dichotomous, will be explored later.

The new idea of a cultural, ideographic science challenged scholars to think about just how precise, unique context-specific evaluations could be produced. It was at this point that 'reflexivity' – so central to contemporary qualitative research – was introduced. Dilthey described the notion of '*verstehen*', which for the first time set out the contribution of the subjectivity of the analyst, which reflected their own experience and led them to a particular perspective or description of the experience being studied (Hughes, 1959). The connection between this debate and current research was secured through the work of Mead and the Chicago school, which gave rise to symbolic interactionism – for qualitative researchers the bedrock for many qualitative approaches (Holloway, 1997). The debate also had practical implications for how the various disciplines that were emerging under the broad umbrella of social sciences organised and conducted themselves and their approach to study. Sociology, psychology and politics divided into two camps – positivist and normative. The positivist school saw themselves as scientists, conducting value-free enquiries, whereas the normative school offered descriptions that raised questions about how things should work.

Weber and the development of sociology

Max Weber (1864–1920) is perhaps the most prominent example of the implications of such separation. 'The object of study for sociology,' he argued, 'is the scientific investigation of the general cultural significance of the socio-economic structure of a human community' (Weber, 1963). Although values of culture could also be a proper route of enquiry, they had a non-rational foundation and consequently a scientific study could not address their validity. However, sociology had a key contribution to make by systematically describing discrepancies between professed values and observed actions. According to Murphy *et al.* (1998), Weber had a profound and lasting influence on the qualitative methods currently in use, and his arguments have been very influential in legitimising qualitative research. One important contribution that he made was to reject the notion that quantification and measurement were the only tools available to a proper scientific enquiry (Freund, 1968; Aron, 1970). Weber himself used quantification extensively, but argued equally that coherent and logically organised systems of concepts could produce a firm enough account of a domain to form the basis for clear interpretation and effective action. Echoes of this insight are seen today. For example, they can be found in an editorial by Sackett *et al.* (1996) allocating quantitative and qualitative research their appropriate places in evidence-based medicine. Even in case studies, Weber used systematic descriptions of unique events in order to elicit some regularities from those events, if not precise laws in the more strict scientific sense. Interpretative understanding, Weber argued, was one means of developing a general science of society (Freund, 1968).

Mill, positivism and the laws of induction

Two years after Kant's death saw the birth of John Stuart Mill (1806–1873), whose philosophy was to develop further some of the arguments laid out by Hume, Berkeley and indeed Kant himself. It is in the work of Mill that we see the first application of the idea of positivism that was introduced by the French philosopher Auguste Comte (1798–1857) in his *Positive Philosophy*. Comte (who also coined the term 'sociology') emphasised the belief that natural science was the most important paradigm and the source of all possible valid knowledge. He expressed the view, typical of that held in the nineteenth century, that the sciences could be seen as a hierarchy, with the basic natural sciences, physics and chemistry at the pinnacle (and in that order), and with those sciences more closely related to the behaviour of societies, institutions and individuals at the bottom, each tier being constrained by the laws of the ones above. Comte's work is considered to be the classical expression of the positivist view, namely that the empirical sciences are the only valid source of knowledge (Comte, 1993). It is important to remember that Comte was developing and publishing these ideas just at the time when Parisian medicine was revisiting many of its institutions and policies, focusing on the importance of precise systematic observations, correlating anatomical findings with clinical presentations and, to all intents and purposes, as a discipline practising the positivist philosophy that he espoused. For the purposes of this chapter, it is the relationship of the sciences in the hierarchy which is important, as it clearly distinguishes in terms of value between those at the top (the natural sciences) and those at the bottom (studies of human relationships and societies).

Murphy *et al.* (1998) argued that positivism, initially described by Comte, developed two distinct strands when used by philosophers on the one hand and by social scientists on the other. For the former it emphasised phenomenalism, which recognised experience as the basis of valid knowledge. For the social sciences it had three implications, all of which retained the notion of the natural sciences as the dominant paradigm (Giddens, 1974). First, there was the implication that the processes and methods of natural science could be adapted to the social sciences. Secondly, the application of positivism in the social sciences was value-free activity. Thirdly, as a result of the first two implications, the outcomes of a social enquiry would have the same characteristics as those of a natural scientific enquiry. Throughout the twentieth century, positivism has dominated social and scientific research. This was a system of enquiry that recognised only observable phenomena, objective relationships, and the laws governing them. The belief that the method of logic upon which the physical sciences were constructed could be applied to the social sciences became one of the central tenets of positivism (Grbich, 1999).

However, according to both Giddens (1974) and Murphy *et al.* (1998), the application of positivism to the social sciences has been threatened by accumulating evidence that the social world is different from the natural world, and the emerging argument that human action is better understood as a creative act of rule orienting, rather than the more deterministic notion of rule following. Central to the notion of positivism was the idea of objectivity, and the relationship between cause and effect. Mill was one of the first to describe the reaction of *effects* upon *causes*: 'the circumstances in which mankind are placed, operating according to their own laws and to the laws of human nature, form the characters of the human beings; but the human beings in their turn mould and shape the circumstances for themselves and for those who come after them' (Mill, 1974). Mill's great contribution was to embed the notion of induction firmly in the social sciences. His sequence – observe, induce, formulate, deduce, hypothesise, test and observe – is his consistent legacy (Fletcher, 1971). Although this has clear parallels with the natural sciences, exactness in the social sciences was always going to be more difficult to achieve, simply because of the inherent complexity of the phenomena involved.

The third period: qualitative research in the twentieth century

The historical origins of contemporary qualitative methods are to be found in the developments in social anthropology that occurred in the years between the two World Wars. Before Malinowski, who really introduced the notion of participant observation in his *Argonauts of the Western Pacific* (Malinowski, 1922), anthropological accounts, mainly from travellers, had lacked context (Urry, 1993). At the turn of the century Haddon introduced and refined fieldwork, taking up the challenge of going directly to traditional societies in person and questioning key informants individually via an interpreter. Fieldwork was further developed by Haddon's colleague Rivers in anthropological studies in Australia and elsewhere, and by Rivers' student Radcliffe Brown (Stalking, 1995).

Although it was Malinowski who did most to develop participant observation in qualitative research, in doing so he still espoused the importance of 'scientific values': 'The results of scientific research in any branch of learning ought to be presented in a manner absolutely candid and above board' (Malinowski, 1922). Some of these emphases are still important today. He distinguished between data obtained from direct observation, data received indirectly through an interpreter, and inferences drawn by a researcher in a summary report (Malinowski, 1922). He also emphasised context, advocating that descriptions of typical events should be accompanied by accounts of the ways of thinking and feeling about those events among the participants. For Malinowski, the goal was 'to grasp the native's point of view, his relation to life, to realise *his* vision of *his* world' (Malinowski, 1922) (his emphasis).

In the 1930s, Malinowski endorsed what became known as mass observation (Mass Observation, 1938). This was a movement which sought to re-democratise politics by asking participants, who were spread nationwide throughout the British Isles, to keep diaries in which they recorded their own daily experiences. It was Malinowski's contribution to the mass observation report that addressed the still delicate tension between subjectivity and objectivity in qualitative research. On the one hand, there is the unique and personal experience of acting in a human society. Social scientists, on the other hand, attempt to observe and record human actions as a clue to these inner processes, document their findings and produce data – in much the same way as science did in natural experiments. In this way, Malinowski said, the subjective behaviour of human beings could become the objective data of the social scientist.

Harrison extended this debate further in *The future of sociology* (Harrison, 1947). He imagined a spectrum of observation, with at one end a philosophical approach which, in his own words, produced laws without observation, and at the other an absorption with quantitative methods which simply satisfied mathematical criteria (Harrison, 1947). Sociology was a potential mediator between these two extreme positions, and could become the 'anthropology of civilised societies' (Harrison, 1947). Harrison took the notion of precise methodologies forward by listing a variety of different types of method, ranging from interviews to observation and what he called penetration, or observation in private settings. The Mass Observation movement, which had been the exemplar of qualitative research in Britain, became increasingly influenced by Government contracts, producing the first qualitative medical sociology report – *Meet Yourself at the Doctor's* – in 1949 (Mass Observation, 1949). Further developments in qualitative methods and social science were delayed until the 1960s, when the incumbent Labour Government demanded more and better social research to inform policy making (Murphy *et al.*, 1998).

Qualitative–quantitative tensions in the twentieth century

At the beginning of the twentieth century, the debates about what constituted 'truth', which the historical description in this section has addressed, focused on two basic approaches to research – qualitative and quantitative. Quantitative researchers assume a singular ontology that is objective, independent and measurable (Brown, 2001). Their epistemological approach, deriving from this, proposes that measurable influences (termed independent variables) affect outcomes (dependent variables) proportionately, as cause and effect. Precise relationships between phenomena can be described by distilling raw numerical data using the conventions of statistics.

Qualitative researchers do not, on the whole, assume a singular ontology. For most of them the notion of 'truth' is not absolute, but rather it resides in gaining an understanding of an individual's frame of reference, by acquiring a detailed knowledge of their views, attitudes and beliefs. The frame of reference thus described is recognised as being socially and historically constructed, and influenced by passing through the researcher's interpretive prism (which is itself socially and historically located) (Denzin and Lincoln, 1994). However, there is considerable variation among qualitative researchers with regard to how one can gain access to 'truth', and it is accepted within qualitative research that one can both create and test hypotheses, and use statistics, to describe the relationship between variables (Grbich, 1999).

Smith and Heshusius (1986) identify three stages in the debate between these two approaches to describing truth, which they term conflict, détente and co-operation. They are each identified with a particular view about the approach to research, which can be described as purist, situationalist or pragmatist (Rossman, 1985). Conflict, Smith and Heshusius argue, was the position for virtually three-quarters of the twentieth century. Characterised by a purist approach to research, qualitative and quantitative techniques were considered to derive from quite different theoretical positions, divided fundamentally by their respective notions of objectivity and subjectivity. However, the last quarter of the twentieth century saw a gradual thawing of this position, with an acceptance that the methodologies could act in parallel. Philosophical differences became submerged in the détente of comparability. This then evolved into a more active co-operation between the two approaches, in which some of the methods of quantitative research could enhance the rigour of qualitative techniques. In the pragmatism of compatibility, the epistemological differences seemed to have become obscured (Grbich, 1999).

But does this desire for pragmatic collaboration between the two approaches work? Several studies in the 1990s have attempted to combine both of these methodologies, either to seek convergence of data, or to produce a fuller explanation of a phenomenon. Although a study by Pradilla (1992) of students' perceptions of their academic supervisors produced broadly consistent results in its quantitative and qualitative arms (and was thus declared to have achieved convergent triangulation), a study by Prein (1992) in the same year did not. That study investigated the links between women's professional careers and their private family biographies. The qualitative approach, using mainly interviews, identified family as the most important factor influencing decisions. However, the quantitative arm, using mainly cluster analysis, identified the particular profession as the dominant influence on decisions. The researchers declared the results completely contradictory (Prein, 1992).

In medicine, the last decade of the twentieth century did see a gradually increasing acceptance of qualitative research processes in a field that had previously been dominated exclusively by quantitative research. Some medical institutions, including grant-awarding bodies, tried to draw up guidelines for qualitative research, in a move that could be interpreted both as legitimising and, at the same time, as constraining the boundaries of such research. Although this has been a welcome development at an institutional level, qualitative researchers in the field still report serious problems with having their research methods understood let alone accepted by senior medical professionals (Sweeney G, 2002, personal communication).

Within the last decade, this debate has been further complicated by an acceptance of the possible limitations of the explanatory model in medicine (Kernick and Sweeney, 2001), and calls for an enquiry into the potential advantages of an explanatory model, predicated on non-linear change, known as complexity, which will be described in detail in the next chapter (Plsek, 2000; Sweeney and Kernick, 2002). The need to consider a revision of medicine's explanatory model, which these papers called for, was heavily influenced by the implications of Heisenberg's uncertainty principle for the notion of accuracy and precision (Sweeney and Griffiths, 2002). At the risk of oversimplifying some complicated mathematics, Heisenberg asserted that the very act of measurement influenced the system that was being measured (Cohen and Stewart, 1994). His quantum state – that is, the combination of velocity and position – could only be approximated. The mechanism of observation determined the observability of a phenomenon, collapsing its other potentialities. This is the basis of the Copenhagen agreement (Cohen and Stewart, 1994). On the face of it, this understanding confronts scientific determinism as applied to social and some physical phenomena, and its implications are still being worked out (Feinstein, 2002; Sweeney and Kernick, 2002). In the second half of the twentieth century, advances in the power of computers led researchers, who were modelling biological systems with increasing accuracy, to recognise the extreme sensitivity of systems to their initial conditions. An understanding began to emerge, which we shall explore shortly, that it was important to understand not just what the structure of a system was, but also how those structural elements related to and interacted with each other (Sweeney and Griffiths, 2002). A reductionist approach to understanding how any system worked was necessary but in itself insufficient (Evans and Sweeney, 1998). While these debates continue, what they seem to imply is that the assumption that any research can capture absolute truth has been seriously undermined.

Summary

Within the naturalistic tradition one discerns the view that, initially, an understanding of the nature of human action could be determined by adopting the same approach as that deployed to acquire scientific knowledge. The origins of this trend can be found in Bacon's writings, and were developed through Descartes' duality and Kant's description of causality. They reached a pinnacle in the hierarchy of knowledge, described by Comte, in which scientific knowledge was placed at the top. Running parallel with, but as a counterpoint to, this hierarchy was the view that the inherent nature of social action is more complex and less predictable than scientific knowledge. The theoretical origins of this viewpoint are found in Berkeley's immaterialism and its relationship to a socially constructed theory of knowledge. Mill's ideas about the impact of effect on antecedent causes represent an important milestone in the development of this trend, which was expressed at the beginning of the twentieth century by Weber's acceptance of the non-rational nature of enquiry into human communities, and his abandonment of quantification as the sole mechanism for proper enquiry. The product of the tension between these two trends was the distinction, much fretted over in the second half of the twentieth century, between quantitative and qualitative approaches. For some – for example, Grbich (1999) – this tension was dissipated in détente, and then methodological co-operation, towards the end of the last century.

Let us reflect on the two traditions discussed so far, namely the scientific tradition from which the contemporary explanatory model in medicine arose, and the naturalistic tradition, providing a different model for observing, recording and interpreting the human predicament. In the previous chapter, exploration of the explanatory model revealed its basis in a particular ontology (a singular reality) and a related epistemology, based upon empiricism and verificationism.

The historical lineage of a naturalistic tradition, described in this chapter, offers a different, complementary view of how the nature of reality might be established, considers another possible ontology, based upon a socially constructed reality, and offers a related epistemological framework, framed in the precepts of qualitative research. If the biomedical tradition expresses a predominantly reductionist world-view, the naturalistic tradition adopts a more relational view, arguing for an understanding not just of the structure of a system, but also of the relationship between the structural components. In the third quarter of the twentieth century, a third intellectual tradition, predicated on non-linear change, emerged from a diverse range of research fields – mainly biology, computing and mathematics. It is termed complexity, and I argue that this could constitute a third tradition, and an extension of the two traditions that have already been described. The next chapter explores this tradition by following, as best as can be done, its historical origins (conscious always of the post-hoc rationality inherent in that kind of analysis), considering the implications of that analysis for clinical medicine, and speculating on a methodology which might allow us to deploy the principles of complexity in contemporary healthcare.

Chapter 5

The non-linear tradition: historical development of complexity

Introduction

This chapter presents the key ideas in the development of complexity, describes the nature of complex adaptive systems, and reflects on how those principles can be applied in healthcare. The term 'system' follows the definition given by Plsek (2000), namely the coming together of parts, their interaction and sense of purpose. Complexity is the term used to describe one of four generic types of dynamic behaviour that a system can exhibit. The first two system behaviours are stasis and order. Stasis denotes the absence of dynamic behaviour, and order denotes a behaviour that is predictable, linear and stereotypical. Chaos refers to a system that appears random, but within which there is determinism and hidden order. Complexity is the dynamic state between order and chaos. Battram (1998) gives the analogy of the breaking surf-wave. The tube in such a large curling wave can be regarded as the complex phase of the wave's behaviour, the phase in the wave's development before it crashes into chaos on the beach. Complexity exists at the edge of chaos.

Three points will be conveyed in this chapter. These are the pervasive nature of non-linear systems, the importance of the interaction between the components of such systems (termed the system's organising relations), and emergence. Emergence denotes the ability of such systems, through the iterative patterning of their interactive relations, to create fresh behaviours and properties, whose nature could not have been predicted simply by understanding the system's components alone. This chapter presents the principal developments of complexity in a chronological sequence in order to build up a picture of the paradigm developing in a wide range of increasingly related disciplines – biology, mathematics, ecology and computing.

The origins of the non-linear paradigm: the debate about structure and pattern

The detail of this historical overview focuses on the twentieth century, when the principles of complexity were first defined, and their potential application in a wide range of disciplines was recognised. The debate, which led to the current detailed understanding of complex systems, began early in the twentieth century among biologists who debated the nature of cell differentiation. However, this debate about the relative importance of structure and pattern in systems was not new. It can be found at the dawn of Western thought, when an enquiry into the relationship between structure (or matter) and pattern (or form) was first recorded by Thales, Parmenides and Pythagoras. Aristotle also recognised the distinction between matter and form. Matter contained the essence of all things, but only as a potentiality, Aristotle argued, and form or pattern was what gave this essence actuality (Sweeney and Griffiths, 2002). The Greeks also struggled with determinism. Was the universe governed by deterministic laws? Can we predict precisely what will happen to systems, and if so, how?

Epicurus set out what became the conventional position at that time, asserting that the world was made up of atoms and a void. The Greeks believed that the atoms fell through the void at the same speed and on parallel paths. This model immediately posed the problem of human freedom. In what could the meaning of human freedom consist if the world was thus deterministically composed of atoms? Epicurus proposed a solution which he termed 'clinamen.' Lucretius described Epicurus' solution as follows:

> *While the first bodies are being carried downwards by their own weight in straight lines through the void, at times quite uncertain and at uncertain places, they deviate slightly from their course, just enough to have been defined as having changed direction.* (Bailey, 1947)

Heraclitus, contributing to this debate, argued that novelty need not be introduced if the nature of *becoming* was emphasised. He argued that 'truth lies in having grasped the essential becoming of nature, that is having represented it as implicitly infinite, as a process in itself' (cited in Popper, 1963). Later, in the *Sophist*, Plato concluded that man needs to incorporate both being and becoming into any explanatory framework, a duality which has tested Western philosophy ever since (Plato, 1979).

To gain a more detailed understanding of how complexity emerged as a valuable way of making sense of the world, it is worth considering the tension between the two schools of biology – vitalism and organicism – at the beginning of the twentieth century.

Early twentieth-century biology: the problem of cell differentiation

Early in the twentieth century, biologists became interested in how cells in living systems were able to differentiate. How could organisms, whose cells multiplied in number from one to two, from two to four, and so on, doubling each time, differentiate if their initial genetic material was identical? How could this identical genetic material produce tissues as diverse as skin, muscle, nerve and bone? Biologists were divided into two schools – vitalism and organicism. Although both were opposed to a simplistic, reductionist understanding of biological systems, they differed markedly in their proposed understanding of cell differentiation. Vitalists thought that an additional non-physical force must be added to the physics and chemistry of the cells to explain their ability to differentiate. The organicists disagreed with this view, arguing that what was important was an understanding of the relationships between the components – what they called their organising relations (Haraway, 1976). In the early decades of the twentieth century the biologist Joseph Woodger and the biochemist Lawrence Henderson made important contributions by introducing the terms 'organising relations' and 'systems thinking', respectively. What Woodger was emphasising by using the term 'organising relations' was the idea that the essence of a system resided not in the structure of each component, but in the way that each component in a system could interact with, relate to and ultimately adapt alongside other components of the system (Capra, 1996). The emergence of systems thinking had a profound influence on scientific thinking generally in the Western world. Its central tenet was that the essential properties of a living system are the properties of the whole, a property held by none of the parts separately (Haraway, 1976). For systems thinking, the context in which any system operated was of fundamental importance.

Heisenberg's uncertainty principle

Developments in physics were informed by and advanced this emerging understanding of complex adaptive systems. Heisenberg's uncertainty principle which, put most simplistically, proposed that the more one measured the velocity of a particle in a system, the less one could accurately determine the location of that particle, and vice versa, had a dramatic effect on the conventional understanding of what 'science' meant. In Heisenberg's own words, 'the foundation of physics has started moving, and this motion has caused the feeling that the ground would be cut from under science' (Heisenberg, 1971). The relevance of this uncertainty principle is elegantly set out by Cohen and Stewart (1994): 'The answers we get', they write, 'depend on the questions we ask.' Consider, as Cohen and Stewart do, the analogy of a tree. We can interrogate the properties of a tree as a plant, or as a boat, or as a pole for holding up telephone lines. The more we know about the tree as a boat, the less we shall understand about its plant properties. The uncertainty principle operates in this context, too. One cannot simultaneously test a tree for its telephone-line-holding properties and its boat-like properties.

Heisenberg was commenting on a shift, as he saw it, from understanding the parts to understanding the whole as part of a general conceptual revolution, so much so that he entitled his biography *Der Tiel und das Ganze – The Part and the Whole* – only to discover that his publishers, failing to realise the subtlety of the title, had renamed the book *Physics and Beyond* (Heisenberg, 1971).

1940s: development of systems theory

Systems theory is conventionally associated with the work of von Bertalanffy, an Austrian biologist whose contribution was to bring together developments in biology, ecology, quantum physics and Gestalt psychology into a new way of thinking which operated in terms of connectedness, relationships and context (von Bertalanffy, 1968). The key characteristics of systems thinking, in relation to living systems, are as follows.

- There is a shift in focus from the parts to the whole.
- The essential properties of living systems are properties of the whole, and none of the parts have these properties.
- These essential properties arise from the organising relationship between the parts.
- These properties are destroyed by reducing the system to its component parts.

- Systems nest within other systems – cellular systems nest within physiological bodily systems, which nest within a human body, which nests within a person.
- At different levels within each living system, there is an increasing degree of complexity. This is described as emergent, as it 'emerges' at different levels within the system.

von Bertalanffy combined these insights from the first half of the twentieth century with the process-oriented philosophy of Whitehead (1929) and with Cannon's (1939) concept of homeostasis to create a theory of open systems. One example of an open system is cellular metabolism – a continuous cyclical process of synthesis, production of nutrients and excretion of waste that occurs within an open environment in terms of its dependency on, and interrelationship with, other provider systems (which provide the material for metabolism) and receiver systems (which receive the metabolic products of that system).

1950s: development of self-organisation

Self-organising behaviour refers to the tendency within complex systems for patterns of observable, coherent behaviour to emerge from what initially appear to be random interactions. This was first observed by two chemists, Belousov and Zhabotinski, in a very simple chemical reaction (which can be easily reproduced). They prepared a mixture of citric acid, sulphuric acid and potassium bromate, placed it in a shallow dish and stirred it. When this is done, bright blue dots appear and spread, and then red dots appear in the centre of the blue dots, forming expanding blue and red rings. When these rings run into each other, they do not superimpose like waves, but form more intricate red and blue circular patterns. This was the first (and is still the most easily reproducible) example of spontaneous formation of patterns from a sea of chaos (Cohen and Stewart, 1994).

One might ask, so what? Self-organising features are emergent properties of complex adaptive systems. They are emergent in the sense that their nature could not have been predicted from a reductionist understanding of the separate constituents of the system. For example, a wave is an emergent property of water. Self-organising behaviour is a fundamental feature of complex adaptive systems. And since complex adaptive systems are pervasive in biological, human and organisational communities, it is important to understand the nature of self-organising behaviour in order to ascertain how those systems work (Cilliers, 1998). Self-organisation operates through positive feedback within a system. In a biological complex system, activity that confers an advantage on the system, or causes it to behave positively, tends to augment the influence of those agents or activities associated with the desired state through positive feedback. Over time, the system will preferentially weight the input of agents whose actions provide positive output, thus establishing repeating patterns of behaviour, which the system expresses as stable characteristics.

Computer specialists were able to reproduce self-organising behaviour in their early modelling of binary systems. Binary systems are systems whose elements can switch on and off, depending on the state of adjacent elements within the systems. While the work was taking place with electrically lit binary computing systems modelling neural activity in the brain, researchers noted the emergence, after a period of random flickering of the lights in the model, of a clear pattern of repeated cycles. Even if the system was started randomly, an ordered pattern would emerge. The process of ordered emergence of coherent behaviour was termed self-organisation (Ashby, 1952). Within a decade of Ashby's report, Heinz von Foerster proposed that in the process of self-organisation, systems increased their internal order (von Foerster and Zoff, 1962), an observation which seemed to counter the second law of thermodynamics. These ideas then gained widespread credibility and found increasingly subtle application in a wide range of fields.

In thermodynamics, the Nobel-Prize-winning work of Prigogine (1998) showed how an open system, far from equilibrium, had the capacity to respond to change and disorder by re-organising itself at a higher level of organisation. Prigogine made a series of observations about entropy, which can be loosely understood as the amount of disorder in a system that is running down. The conventional, Newtonian view was that the amount of entropy was increasing. That was the basis for his Newton's second law of thermodynamics. However, Prigogine measured not just the amount of entropy in a system but what happened to it. He found that deterioration in systems was not inevitable. The disruption or disequilibrium in a system, associated with entropy, need not inevitably lead to dissipation (or equilibrium, the equivalent of dynamic death). Prigogine used the term 'dissipative structures' to describe those systems which could give up their original structures to recreate themselves in new forms. Such systems, according to Prigogine, had the ability to self-organise.

Self-organisation became a central plank of the explanatory model in other fields. The Gaia hypothesis of the English biochemist Lovelock, and the Chilean neurophysiologists Maturana and Varella, all incorporate the notion of self-organisation in their explanations (Capra, 1996).

Developments in mathematics: self-reinforcing feedback and non-linear equations

Parallel developments in mathematics and quantum physics fuelled the development of this non-linear paradigm. Towards the end of the nineteenth century, mathematics had two sets of tools for solving problems, namely deterministic equations and statistical analysis, for simple and complicated systems, respectively. Both shared the key feature of linearity, of which the equation

$$y = x + 1$$

is the simplest example.

Geometry, which was the original approach to mathematical solutions originating in Greece, and algebra, which was introduced several hundred years later by the Persians, had been unified by Descartes' analytical geometry, by which technique mathematicians were able to represent linear equations pictorially, using Cartesian coordinates in graphical form. Newton's subsequent contribution was to develop differential calculus, which allowed mathematicians to represent the motion of a body that was undergoing acceleration. What mathematicians in the early twentieth century found, however, was that the exact solutions provided by the elegant Newtonian mathematics applied to relatively few simple systems in real life. Their dilemma was best illustrated by their failure to solve the problem of three celestial bodies under mutual gravitational attraction (Stewart, 1989).

Stewart (1989) illustrates the conspicuous tendency of mathematicians to linearise their equations and thus the solutions they could provide: 'it was a linear world for most of the nineteenth and twentieth century.' However, in the second half of the twentieth century there was a gradual acceptance in mathematics of the predominance of non-linear systems in nature. What mathematicians found when they applied their equations to non-linear phenomena was striking. Simple deterministic equations produced rich and unexpected solutions. Exact prediction, it seemed, was impossible, and self-reinforcing feedback appeared to exert an important influence on such systems (Capra, 1996). In non-linear systems, small changes could have dramatic effects as they could be amplified by self-reinforcing feedback. A simple example will show this fundamental characteristic of non-linear systems.

Mathematically, a feedback loop consists of a process referred to as iteration – that is, repetitive solving of an equation, feeding back the previous solution to the same function to obtain an iterated new solution, and repeating this process over and over again. So if the function is to multiply the variable y by 4, shown by the statement $f(y) = 4y$, then the iteration consists of repeated multiplications of that function:

$$y \rightarrow 4y$$

$$4y \rightarrow 16y$$

$$16y \rightarrow 64y$$

and so on.

A very simple iteration in non-linear mathematics which illustrates this key idea of non-linearity is derived from multiple (iterative) solving of the simple function

$$y \rightarrow ky(1 - y)$$

where y lies between 0 and 1. Consider iterative solutions to this function where $k = 3$, and y lies between 0 and 1. This can be worked out easily on a hand calculator, but below I present a few solutions which show non-linear change.

Where $y = 0$ $0 \rightarrow 0(1 - 0) = 0$
Where $y = 0.2$ $0.2 \rightarrow 0.6(1 - 0.2) = 0.48$
Where $y = 0.4$ $0.4 \rightarrow 1.2(1 - 0.4) = 0.72$
Where $y = 0.6$ $0.6 \rightarrow 1.8(1 - 0.6) = 0.72$
Where $y = 0.8$ $0.8 \rightarrow 2.4(1 - 0.8) = 0.48$
Where $y = 1$ $1 \rightarrow 3(1 - 1) = 0$

The numbers stretch out and then fold over, coming back to zero, in what is known as the Baker transformation (Briggs and Peat, 1989). Importantly, mathematicians pointed out that linearity was a subset of non-linearity – that is, a special case of the simple non-linear equation

$$y = ax^n + c$$

where a is a constant and $n = 1$.

A seminal contribution to the mathematics of complexity was made by the work of mathematician and scientist Henri Poincare, who reintroduced pictorial representation into mathematics with his topological geometry, a technique whereby non-linear systems could actually be drawn as they evolved. Poincare was interested in how systems evolved from the perspective of the whole, rather than by considering the parts of the system in isolation. He theorised about the generic relationship of the whole of science to the facts of which it is composed: 'Science is built up with facts, just as a house is built with stones. But a collection of facts is no more science than a heap of stones is a house' (Poincare, 1952). In a later essay he writes, 'The aim of science is not things in themselves . . . but the relation between things; outside these relations there is no reality knowable' (Poincare, 1958).

The application of mathematics to non-linear biological systems

Developments in the mathematics of non-linear systems initially improved researchers' understanding of thermal and fluid dynamics (Gribbin, 2004). The relevance of such mathematics to biological systems was subsequently explored, resulting in the ability to model the evolution of relationships between predators and prey In defined ecological systems, such as a forest. For the purposes of the arguments that are being developed in this book, it is worthwhile reflecting on the nature of this modelling, as it was later applied to the spread of infectious diseases, and it still holds out considerable potential as a research tool for modelling other clinical conditions (Holt, 2002a).

Consider, in order to preserve clarity in the explanatory principles, a simple exploration of the evolution of a population of insects, where the entire population dies off in the winter, after laying eggs that will hatch out to provide the next generation in the following season. We start with a population of x individuals, each of which (again for ease of mathematical modelling) produces an average of B offspring. We take into account the fact that some insects will die before producing offspring – for example, if the initial numbers are large, and there is not enough food for all the population members. This is accounted for by setting an upper limit for the population, which can be done quite accurately (Cohen and Stewart, 1994), and then calculating the actual number, x, as a fraction of this, such that x will always lie between 0 and 1. Then, to take into account premature deaths, the growth factor, Bx, is multiplied by $(1 - x)$ in a process termed renormalisation.[3]

We can then say that the population of such a system will rise and fall as a function of the birth rate, B. This is calculated, for varying values of B, by iterating the following equation:

$$x(\text{next}) = Bx(1 - x).$$

This is a non-linear equation, as it multiplies out to:

---

[3] This works because if the population level at the outset of the analysis is very low, all of the insects will survive, $(1 - x)$ will approximate to 1, and so the growth rate will be almost exactly Bx. Conversely, if the initial population level is high, x will nearly equal 1, and $(1 - x)$ will approximate to 0, reflecting the fact that many members of the population will starve or be eaten by predators.

$$Bx - Bx^2.$$

The equation will also involve feedback, as the output from the first iteration will be the input to calculate the next step, or generation.

It is interesting, in terms of the application of non-linear mathematics to living systems, to see what happens to the predicted population of insects when the value of B varies. Consider the following few examples. When B is less than 1, the population will die out, whatever the starting value of x. When B is greater than 1, but less than 3, this logistic equation settles down, after a sufficiently large number of iterations (that is, in real terms, generations), to a fairly constant population, with the equation solving itself at around 0.66, whatever value of x between 0 and 1 is applied. This indicates a population that is fairly steadily settled at around two-thirds of its maximum number. When B is greater than 3, something quite different happens.

Once the iteration of this equation has been solved enough times, with values of B just greater than 3, two different constant levels of population emerge, one with a high population level and the other with a relatively low population level. In real terms this makes sense. In one year there may be a large population, which eats all of the food, and many individuals starve and die without reproducing. The next generation therefore has a smaller population with plenty of food. They all survive and lay eggs, so that the next generation is larger, and so on. This phenomenon is known as period doubling, when a system moves from a single equilibrium to a two-cycle steady state. Such an iterative calculation of population levels can be continued. When the value of B (indicating the average number of offspring) is equal to 3.44, the period doubling of the system moves from 2 to 4, and it jumps again, from 4 to 8, when the value of B is equal to 3.56. When the value of B exceeds 4, there is no pattern to the cycle, and the value of x, the total population, dots about randomly. This is chaos, and it has been extensively studied (Tennison, 2002). It has been reached through the iterative solving of a deterministic non-linear equation exposed to self-referential feedback. This conjunction of determinism and positive feedback, with repeated iterations leading to unpredictability, is characteristic of chaos (Gleick, 1998).

For mathematicians, the next step, which generated a huge amount of interest in this type of mathematical modelling, was the calculation of the interval between period doubling – that is, the numerical distance in the system between period 1, fairly steady state, and period 2, oscillation between high and low, then period 4, then period 8. Working at Los Alamos Laboratory in New Mexico, the mathematician Mitchell Feigenbaum calculated that the period interval between each bifurcation occurred at a constant ratio, namely 1:4.669. Researchers in other fields soon discovered that this ratio, known as Feigenbaum's number, applies to any such self-referential system (that is, one which feeds back into itself via regular iterations), whether it occurs in biology, electrical circuits, geological systems, oscillating chemical reactions or even, in principle, the business cycle of the economy. Feigenbaum's number appears to be a universal constant, applied to any such iterating self-referential system where period doubling occurs, in literally any domain (Cohen and Stewart, 1994; Gleick, 1998; Gribbin, 2004). I shall return to the potential importance of Feigenbaum's number when speculating about the implications of non-linear mathematics in clinical medicine.

Feigenbaum's constant is related to another visible feature of self-referencing systems which exhibit period doubling. This is the *pattern* of doubling, which can be charted at various stages in the system's evolution. When we see, at the outset, the first period doubling cycle, we can visualise the system bifurcating so that it diagrammatically resembles a tuning fork. As the system moves from a two-cycle period to a four-cycle period, this bifurcation shape is reproduced, in smaller and smaller iterations, as shown in Figure 5.1. The point at stake here is the self-similarity of the repeated patterning of these bifurcations. This patterning, known as fractal patterning, is characteristic of chaotic systems.

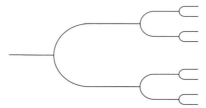

Figure 5.1 Fractal patterning in period-doubling systems.

In the same way that Feigenabum's number is a universal constant, fractal patterning has been found in all chaotic systems, and has been extensively researched in analogue telephone signals, thermodynamics, geology, biology, the music of Bach and the paintings of Jackson Pollock, the American abstractionist, (Casti, 1995).

1960s: Lorenz Butterfly and the sensitivity to initial conditions

Advances in computing during the third quarter of the twentieth century allowed scientists to explore the nature of complex systems in more and more detail. When exploring non-linear equations, especially equations with several variables which were solved simultaneously, it became clear that the most minute difference in the value of one of the variables at the beginning of a computation could make a huge difference as those equations were solved iteratively, as one would do in order to describe mathematically the evolution of a complex system over time. The classic example of this is found in early attempts to model weather patterns.

In 1963, Edward Lorenz explored how weather systems might be modelled mathematically to determine the extent to which the behaviour of such complex systems could be predicted. He created a model of a simplified atmosphere using just three variables which seemed to be crucial, namely the intensity of air movement, the temperature difference between ascending and descending air currents, and the temperature gradient between the top and the bottom of the atmosphere.

These can be visualised as the three axes of a three-dimensional graph. For each moment in time, one can plot a single point representing the combined functions of the three variables. One can then imagine plotting serial points, showing the location of the simplified atmosphere as time proceeds. Thus the development of weather can be imagined as a tracing out of the single points over time.

Lorenz ran a series of equations, plotting each of these variables over time, and substituting slightly different values for each of the variables as he progressed (Lorenz, 1963). Plotting the results in a notional three-dimensional graph on his computer, he produced the eponymous graph with two lobes, shown in Figure 5.2. This is sometimes referred to as an 'attractor', a term which indicates a representation of the behaviour of a complex system over time (Battram, 1998).

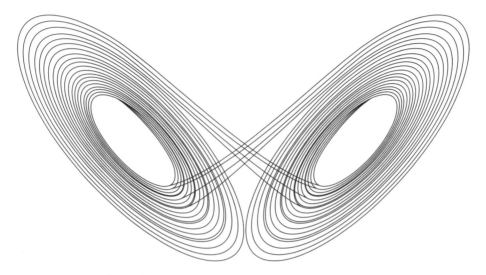

Figure 5.2 Lorenz butterfly.

Lorenz modelling revealed the inherent impossibility of predicting anything other than over a very short range. The tiniest alteration in one of the values – for example, changing a value at the third or fourth decimal place – could have a dramatic effect on the direction of the system, as that result was re-introduced into the modelling equations time and time again. Complex systems, it appeared, were extremely sensitive to their initial conditions. If one tries to string together a set of short-term predictions to create a long-term prediction, tiny errors creep in, and these tiny errors, repeated iteratively as the modelling equations are run, build in much larger errors (Stewart, 1989). However, the overall shape of the Lorenz attractor also implied that the system – in this case broad patterns of weather – will always remain somewhere within those boundaries. Thus one can predict that given a broad set of initial conditions – British summer, say – the weather is unlikely to produce temperatures below freezing or above 40 degrees centigrade. However, it is much more difficult to say precisely what the weather pattern will be in one location at a particular time.

Although it is beyond the scope of this book to explore in detail the mathematical modelling of complex meteorological systems, it should be noted that a firm mathematical basis has been established for analysing the nature and evolution of such systems through, for example, the calculation of Lyapunov exponents. A positive Lyapunov exponent is characteristic of chaotic systems, and confirms that the system under analysis is sensitive to its initial conditions (Schaffer, 1985).

Characteristics of complex systems

At this point we can summarise the key features of complex systems, before going on to consider some examples of them in a range of disciplines.

Five key features can be identified:

1 sensitivity to initial conditions
2 complex responsive processes
3 self-organisation
4 adaptation (leading to co-evolution)
5 emergence.

Sensitivity to initial conditions

Lorenz's work on weather systems demonstrated that, in order to understand how a complex system might evolve, it is crucial to know as much as possible about the initial conditions under which it begins to operate. Lorenz showed that even a tiny alteration in the initial state of one variable in a complex system with a large number of variables (e.g. a weather front) can lead, through self-reinforcing feedback, to large alterations in the way that the system evolves.

The sensitivity of a system to its initial conditions is important because of the nature of the feedback, both positive and negative, which influences the direction that a complex system will take. In the conventional understanding of linear models, the notion of negative feedback, leading to the 'desired' state of equilibrium, dominates descriptions of complex systems. Examples in clinical medicine include the effect of increased levels of thyroid hormone in feeding back to the secretion of thyroid-stimulating hormone, to maintain equilibrium, or the ability of insulin – whether injected, stimulated or secreted from the pancreas – to equilibrate the blood sugar level. However, such biological systems operate with positive as well as negative feedback. Thus, for example, in diabetes there is not simply a failure of negative feedback. The system (that is, the patient) is unable to detect swings in blood glucose levels, is unable to respond to those swings when they occur, and is, during episodes of flux, prone to behaviour which reinforces the direction of change of blood sugar level (away from normal) through lethargy, inattention, and missed or inaccurate dosing of insulin. Thus the system is 'encouraged' to move towards even greater disequilibrium. It is more useful to consider homeostasis as the delicate balancing of a range of inputs, each of which may act on others, rather than as a negative feedback system leading to equilibrium. Holt (2002a) gives the analogy of balancing a snooker cue on the palm of the hand – corrections to a potential imbalance are not undertaken in the plane of the imbalance (the linear response), but by small, repeated corrections in a wide range of directions.

In human systems, the equivalent of the sensitivity to initial physical conditions that was described in relation to weather systems is termed enabling framework or receptive context (Mitelton-Kelly, 2003; Durie et al., 2004). The term evokes the idea of an infrastructure of communicability – a set of conditions that have the potential to facilitate the development of complex conversations and actions whose patterning can, over time, constitute a complex system. Thus a receptive context implies a potentiality for coherent action, a set of values through which coherent action can be expressed, the presence of leadership to initiate complex responsive processes, and the potential to engage other agents to co-create and adapt the system. The evidence from one national study of healthcare organisations undergoing transformation change (Durie *et al.*, 2004) has identified a number of characteristics of receptive context. These include the following: a recognition that ways of working need to be improved, and that within the process of improvement, work practices may become quite different; a recognition that, in order to co-create new, different working practices, relationships are crucial, implying the need both to reconfigure existing relationships and to create new ones; and a recognition, as a consequence of the first two characteristics, that communication is the bedrock for initiating such change, and that within communication the use of language (professional versus informal, and specialist versus lay) is central.

Complex responsive processes

The basic unit of activity within a human complex adaptive system is the communication between individuals through which those individuals co-create and, in the process, make sense of the system. The basic unit of communication is called a complex responsive process (Stacey, 2001). Through their patterning, the system self-organises and develops its unique characteristics. 'The modelling of complex systems', Stacey (2001) asserts, 'demonstrates the possibility that inter-action between entities, each entity responding to others on the basis of its own organising principles, will produce coherent patterns with the potential for novelty in certain conditions.' Stacey maintains that interaction through complex communication constitutes a self-organising process, with coherence (an epi-phenomenon) as one of its emergent properties: 'There is no reason to look for some kind of underlying blueprint, plan or predetermined mechanism other than the interaction itself to explain coherence in human action, with its character-istics of continuity and potential transformation' (Stacey, 2001).

Three points need to be emphasised. First, complex responsive processes have the potential to be transformational (Stacey, 2001). In participating in a complex responsive process, the conversation is changed, each participant is changed, the nature of their relationship can change and, by a ripple effect, the nature of the participants' relationship with the larger system changes. Secondly, these processes are inherently unpredictable. During their course one participant issues a gesture, which in turn calls forth a response from the other, in an iterative, interactive and self-organising process. Thirdly, the patterning of such processes and relationships, formed as a result, constitutes the self-organised characteristics of the system, which confer a degree of stability, allowing it to be recognised and described (Stephenson, 2004). This description of complex responsive processes has two implications for any methodology that purports to analyse a complex system (e.g. a healthcare organisation). First, it should alert researchers to the importance of collating data about relationships – precisely who talks to whom, where (not just formally but via the shadow organisation), and how those discussions develop. Secondly, following on from this, is the recognition that storytelling and narratives become a key data source, as it is within narratives that participants in a system describe their formal and informal participation via conversations. They can recount how these conversations changed the storyteller, and how the system might have changed as a result. This is the approach now adopted by some organisational analysts, particularly those dealing with the transformation of large international companies (Snowden, 2002; Mitelton-Kelly, 2003; Health Complexity Group, 2004).

Self-organisation

The essence of a complex adapting system is located in the basic interaction between each of its agents. This interaction occurs at a one-to-one level, and is then magnified through the interaction of other agents, all of whom interact with each other, either directly or indirectly, through the process of adaptation or co-evolution. Thus the behaviour of complex systems consists of this myriad of local interactions, the patterning of which constitutes the system's behaviour, allowing it to be recognised and described. This process of co-creating coherent patterns of behaviour is called self-organisation. Because complex systems exhibit non-linear behaviour, the nature of such self-organising patterns cannot be predicted precisely, and thus the product of such patterned behaviour – the emergent properties of the system – cannot be anticipated either.[4] Examples of self-organising behaviour include the flocking of birds and the behaviour of the stock market (Battram, 1998). 'Flocking' is the self-organising process created by a group of birds travelling together, and the resultant 'flock' is its emergent property. It is an epi-phenomenon, neither planned in advance nor knowingly constructed in a conscious, concerted effort by the agents (the birds).

Adaptation and co-evolution

Detailed studies of a wide range of ecosystems show clearly that relationships between living organisms are, at their root, co-operative, characterised by coexistence and interdependence (Capra, 1983). Although this view seriously challenges the conventional Darwinian view of evolution, it is supported by a wealth of evidence demonstrating the interplay of adaptation and creation in the process of evolution. Kauffman (1993) illustrates this point by drawing the analogy of a small forest-based ecosystem containing flies, frogs, fish and bears. There are many ways in which the frogs, who want to eat flies, and the flies, who do not want to be eaten, interact. Frogs might develop longer or stickier tongues. Flies might develop more slippery bodies to avoid capture, or an unpleasant taste to deter frogs when they are captured. In a stable state, each of the frogs will eat a proportion of flies each season – but this is a dynamic equilibrium, not a static state. Suppose that a frog does develop a stickier tongue, and is able to catch more flies. At first a larger proportion of flies will be eaten. However, the ones that aren't eaten are likely to be the ones with the gene for a more slippery body, so that this advantage spreads throughout the population of flies, just as the gene for a stickier tongue will spread through the population of frogs. As a result, the system will settle down to a new state, where roughly the same proportion of flies are eaten by the frogs. Although it may appear from the outside as if nothing has changed, there has been a shift in the nature of each of the agents in the system. And although each of the participants has changed, so too has the nature of their interaction, the stickier tongue succeeding in catching the even more slippery body. This is like the 'Red Queen effect' in Lewis

---

[4] However, both can be described.

Carroll's *Through the Looking Glass*, where the Red Queen has to run as fast as she can in order to stay in the same place.[5]

Emergence

Emergence is the key idea that holds together and unifies complex systems. It is an epi-phenomenon, a higher-order feature of complex systems created by the patterning of the interaction of its agents. The term refers to the potential within complex systems, given appropriate initial conditions, to develop behaviours (through self-organisation and co-evolution) which create emergent properties, the nature of which could not have been predicted by knowing the components of the systems at the beginning (the conventional reductionist approach). Emergence is the product of self-organisation. Thus a wave is an emergent property of water, a flock is the emergent property of birds flying together (Battram, 1998), and temperature and pressure are emergent properties of trillions of gas molecules in a box (Tennison B, 2004, personal communication).

Kauffman (1993), a theoretical biologist, has shown in a simple experiment that complexity itself is an emergent property of complex systems. Kauffman invites us to consider a system of a large number of buttons (say around 10 000), laid out on a floor, which are increasingly connected simply by tying them together with thread. You choose a pair of buttons at random and tie them together. Repeat the process, not worrying if you choose, at random, a button that is already attached to another one, as will increasingly happen as you proceed. As the process continues, some buttons will become attached to more than one other button, or to more than two or three others, and finally to more than several hundred others (the vertical axis in Figure 5.3). Each button represents a node in the system – that is, a point to which connections are connected. Each such cluster of buttons can be termed a component of the network. The number of buttons in the largest cluster (the largest component, which may sustain 200–300 connections) is a measure of how complex the system has become. Once the number of connections exceeds half the number of nodes (the thread/button ratio, shown in the horizontal axis in Figure 5.3), it very rapidly changes from one state (a large number of buttons with few connections) to another one (a state in which almost every button is part of the network). This relationship can be plotted quite precisely, as Figure 5.3 shows.

The relevance of emergence to living systems is well described by Gribbin (2004) through the notion of autocatalysis. This term refers to a system that develops the ability to continue to renew and generate itself, and it has been postulated, again by the complexity theorist Stuart Kauffman, as a model to explain the origin of biological life on earth (the model is speculative at present, but is supported by a good deal of circumstantial evidence) (Gribbin, 2004). Imagine, in the primordial chemical broth which existed shortly after the earth's formation, that there developed some chemical substances which acted as catalysts for other substances, like the catalytic process in the Belousov–Zhabotinski reaction referred to on p. 64. Suppose that chemical A catalyses the production of chemical B. As the system develops, chemical B catalyses the

---

[5] Indeed, the term 'Red Queen effect' was introduced into evolutionary biology by Leigh van Valen at the University of Chicago in the 1970s.

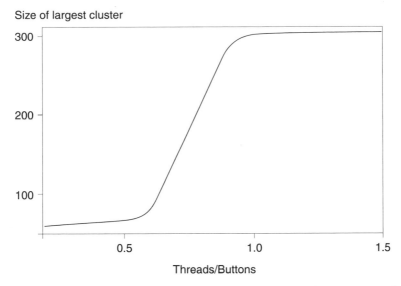

Size of largest cluster

Threads/Buttons

Figure 5.3 Phase transition and the emergence of complexity in a basic connected system.

production of C, and chemical C catalyses the production of D, and so on. If, somewhere down the line of catalytic reactions, chemical X catalyses the production of chemical A, the loop becomes self-generating and autocatalytic. According to Gribbin (2004), Kauffman presents this model, with supportive but not yet definitive evidence, as analogous to the connected-button model, namely as a phase transition in a chemical system involving a sufficient number of connections between the chemicals (analogous to the nodes in the button model). This process of chemical autocatalysis is valuable because it illustrates the idea of connectedness – the crucial interaction of individual components within a system, whose iterative patterning forms a self-organising process with the potential to create emergent properties.

Describing and recognising complex systems

At present there is no firm consensus about what constitutes the necessary and sufficient conditions for a complex and adaptive system to be said to be present. Current opinion (Mitelton-Kelly, 2004; Plsek P, 2004, personal communication) suggests that the identification of a receptive context is a sine qua non, without which there are no grounds to favour the patterning of complex responsive processes or the self-organising of the system. Thus, contemporary experts agree, the absence of receptive context implies that a system will be incapable of co-evolving and will, as a consequence, fall to develop any emergent properties by which it might be recognised, described and explored. This analysis also implies the existence of a temporal relationship between the features of complex systems described above. If the presence of a receptive context is the necessary initiating feature, then in human systems it is the enactment of complex responsive processes which is the next sequential step. In an evolving complex adaptive system, the patterning of such complex responsive processes will lead to self-organisation and, in turn, to the likelihood of co-evolution. Finally, in the evolutionary sequence of a developing complex system, the pattern of self-organisation and co-evolution may lead to the appearance of emergent properties, which tend to be stabilising features of such systems, allowing them to be characterised and recognised – and researched (Stephenson, 2004).

As we shall see, this will have important consequences for researching such systems. Although there is no agreement as to which of the features must be present for a system to be said to be complex and adaptive, one can assume that, in organisational research, for example, the absence of a receptive context is sufficient grounds for asserting that the system under observation could not be complex and adaptive. However, there is no consensus as to whether some or all of the other four features described above need to be present. I speculate that it would be premature to describe a system as complex and adaptive in the absence of clear evidence of complex responsive processes, together with their patterning in clearly identifiable self-organised entities. If a system had evolved to such an extent that it had self-organised, then I take the view that, assuming the continuing presence of a receptive context, co-evolution would be more likely to occur than not. Thus the minimum conditions under which one could describe a system as complex and adaptive would need to have evidence of a receptive context, complex responsive processes and self-organisation. In the next chapter I shall discuss a research methodology that incorporates an understanding of complexity, scrutinising qualitative data in a second-level analysis from a complexity perspective. In this chapter I use the criteria of a complex and evolving system set out above.

1980s to the present: applications of non-linearity in organisations

In the last two decades there has been increasing interest in the application of the principles of complex systems to organisational change both in the commercial sector (Stacey, 2000; Wheatley, 2000) and in healthcare (Plsek, 2000).

Applications in the commercial world

Wheatley (2000) contextualises her interpretation of complexity for organisational change consistently within the intellectual developments described above. She cites Prigogine's understanding of self-organisation and its classic illustration through the Belousov–Zhabotinsky reaction. She echoes Poincare's view that 'relationships are not just interesting, they are all there is to reality' (Wheatley, 2000). Her interpretation of the principles of complexity is informed by quantum physics. Quantum physicists could identify a range of subatomic particles, Wheatley explained, but these could not truly be understood in isolation. They were particles in an intermediate state sustained within a network of interactions (Zukav, 1979). 'Physicists can plot the probability and results of these interactions, but no particle can be drawn independent from the others', she observes (Wheatley, 2000).

Wheatley brings these notions together in a new model of change management predicated on relational dynamics. She cites examples of her own fieldwork in large commercial companies, where the reinterpretation of the principles of complexity has been associated with large-scale successful transformational change. Oticom, the Scandinavian manufacturer of hearing aids, reorganised their head-office space using self-organisation as its guiding principle, in what amounted to a major de-structuring of their entire corporation (Pinchot and Pinchot, 1996). In an attempt to respond more swiftly and flexibly to the changing environment in which they operated, Oticom employees literally gave up their office space and furniture, swapping these for mobile essentials – a cell phone, laptop computer, and file cart on wheels. So did the chief executive, who located himself in marketing, finance or HR, depending on where an immediate need had arisen (Pinchot and Pinchot, 1996).

Buckman Laboratories, a US-based manufacturer of speciality chemicals, have reported an increased commercial capacity following their revised open distrib-uted approach to information – a prerequisite, according to Wheatley, for effective self-organisation. The company recognised that information flow could act as an organisational glue, encouraging richer connectivity between the agents in their system – their employees – and they therefore introduced a company intranet. One of the company's employees, challenged by some tech-nical information that was needed to close a business deal, made use of the recently developed company intranet to request advice. Within hours he received a range of replies from the company's centres in six countries. Not only did this information help him to secure the deal, but also his technical query spawned a further conversation between some of the respondents about the query, which grew into an ongoing conversational resource – an interesting example of self-organisation (Willett, 1999).

Stacey diagram

Ralph Stacey, an organisational development specialist, has explored the application of complexity principles in management theory. One particular contribution that he has made is the agreement certainty matrix shown in Figure 5.4 (Stacey, 2000). In this notional matrix the vertical axis represents *agreement* – that is, agreement about the attributes of a system, and agreement between the agents about an issue arising within that system. *Certainty*, repre-sented by the horizontal axis, is an indication of how sure one can be about the cause-and-effect linkages within the system. Where one is close to certainty, one can usually draw on previous experience of a similar issue in the past. New or unexpected situations locate the agents far from certainty – towards the right of this horizontal line.

This visual matrix can help managers to choose which approach might be best suited to address issues which they can, by reflecting on their attributes, 'locate' at different places within the notional space. For example, when operating in the linear or simple zone, classic rational strategies such as process engineering can be effective. However, in the zone of chaos they will not help. Here it is best to look for patterns by continuously communicating with other agents in the system before applying any coherent strategy. However, it is in the zone of complexity that most of the issues facing large organisations lie. Building networks, enhan-cing communication, working collectively and allowing direction to emerge are the guiding management principles here (Wheatley, 2000).

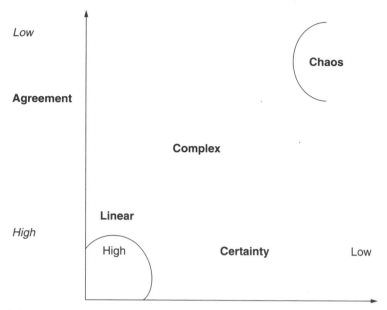

Figure 5.4 Stacey agreement certainty matrix.

Applications in clinical care and healthcare policy

Plsek has recently incorporated the principles of complex adaptive systems into his vision of how the US healthcare system should develop in the twenty-first century. Like Wheatley and Stacey, Plsek focuses on the importance, in healthcare systems, of the connections and interactions between components of the system. 'A healthcare system' he writes, 'is a macro-system. It consists of numerous micro-systems (doctors' offices, hospitals, pharmacies and so on) that are linked to provide comprehensiveness of care.' Plsek distinguishes between mechanical and adaptive systems:

> *In mechanical systems, we can predict what the system will do in great detail. In complex adaptive systems, the parts (which in a healthcare system include human beings) have the ability to respond to stimuli in fundamentally unpredictable ways. For this reason, emergent creative behaviour is a real possibility.* (Plsek, 2000)

Plsek concludes that complexity provides a new paradigm to guide an understanding of how systems work in healthcare.

Within the UK healthcare system, the principles of complex adaptive systems have been reframed by Fraser *et al.* (2003) within the notion of 'agility'. An agile system is one that can respond rapidly to a changing environment and markets. The importance of rich interaction – a key feature of complex adaptive systems – is stressed, as agile commercial organisations draw on their relationships with suppliers, partners and customers to improve their practices. Using flexible working patterns and virtual teaming, agile companies can, it is asserted, deliver products more swiftly, with better quality and at lower cost.

The principles of agility, set out in Box 5.1, strongly evoke the key characteristics of complex adaptive systems, namely receptive context, self-organisation and co-evolution. In the UK there are examples in the NHS where these principles of agility have been applied to healthcare organisations – for example, in the redesign of older people's services in London.

Box 5.1 Attributes of agile systems applied to healthcare

Rapid changeover (e.g. in the use of operating theatres)
Doing today's work today (the basis of advanced access in general practice)
Co-operative rescheduling carried out with partners, stakeholders, patients and carers
Flexibility, particularly in the constitution of teams
Synchronised scheduling
Care coordinated around a specific patient, not as part of mass customisation

(Adapted from Yarrow *et al.*, 2003)

Complexity and clinical medicine

Clinicians in medicine have also been slowly responding to the explanatory potential of this non-linear relational paradigm. Non-linear systems have been proposed as a better basis for understanding physiological and pathological states in infectious diseases (Schaffer, 1985), cardiology (Goldberger and West, 1987), neurology (Holland, 1998) and diabetes (Holt, 2002a). I shall discuss these examples in more detail in Chapter 8.

Moving away from the purely clinical level, non-linear models have also been postulated for education of healthcare professionals (Fraser and Greenhalgh, 2001), for understanding organisational change (Plsek and Wilson, 2001) both in the NHS (Kernick, 2002) and in the North American healthcare system (Zimmerman and Plsek, 1998), and for understanding the development and embedding of clinical governance at the level of primary care trusts (Sweeney and Mannion, 2002; Sweeney, 2003a). Hassey (2002) has proposed a theoretical model for understanding the consultation in general practice, based on the non-linear principles of complexity.

Distinguishing between complex and chaotic systems

Both the Baker transformation and the non-linear equations that are the basis of period doubling systems help to distinguish between chaotic and complex systems. Chaos is concerned with those forms of complexity in which emergent order coexists with disorder (Gleick, 1998). When a system moves from a state of order away from equilibrium towards disorder, a new pattern of order can emerge. This is what lies at the basis of the apparent paradox of order coexisting with disorder, with determinism giving rise to unpredictability through iteration and positive feedback.

Chaos theory is not the same as complexity, and it is helpful to distinguish between the two, particularly in relation to social systems. Chaos theory describes non-linear dynamics based on the iteration of mathematical formulae which, as we have seen with the modelling of biological populations, can give rise to unpredictable behaviour and the intricate patterning of fractals. However, it is within the repeated iteration of the constant formula that the inherent difference between chaotic and complex systems lies. Complex systems may be capable of adapting and evolving, and of changing the rules of their interaction – for example, in relation to a major change in their environment. They are not created simply by the iterative application of a formula. Thus one speaks more of complexity when discussing human systems, as human behaviour allows for choice, and the subsequent alteration of the nature of interaction – it does not mimic mathematical algorithms (Mitelton-Kelly, 2003).

Summary

This chapter has described how in the twentieth century an intellectual tradition predicated on non-linear relational dynamics evolved. Based upon observations in biology, and assisted enormously by advances in mathematics and computer modelling, complexity now presents itself as another explanatory model. This chapter has laid out the key features of complex systems – sensitivity to initial conditions (receptive context in human systems), self-organisation, co-evolution and emergence – and has introduced the notion of period doubling in systems, which can be described using self-referencing logistic equations. Two points still need to be emphasised. First, there is sufficient evidence at present to allow us to state that complex systems are ubiquitous. Secondly, they reflect the importance of non-linear dynamics and organising relationships. The basic unit of activity in a complex system involving human action is the complex responsive process, the iterative patterning of which provides the system, over time, with its self-organising capability and potential for novelty. Emergence is the unifying feature of such systems, and refers to the properties co-created by the interaction of the components of the system in a deterministic but unpredictable way.

The application of the principles of complex adaptive systems is now to be found in a wide range of disciplines, including ecology, thermodynamics, meteorology, chemistry, and more recently management theory and clinical medicine. Such a non-linear paradigm reflects a relational ontology, and constructs its epistemological framework around the principles of complex adaptive systems. Thus the description of complexity in this chapter contributes to the propositions that are unfolding in this book by providing evidence of a third explanatory model.

With regard to clinical medicine, there are two features of complexity that demand serious reflection. These are the paradoxical juxtaposition of determinism and unpredictability, and the notion of complex responsive processes.

The analysis of the iterative patterning of non-linear equations introduced the possibility of bifurcation – the possibility that a system could exhibit widely swinging properties depending on the conditions present at the start of any iteration. Remember what happened to our population of insects. We know that their population will increase and decrease as a function of a fairly simple non-linear equation, but that as the birth rate ('B', the multiplier in the equation) just exceeds 3, two different constant levels of population arose. Further bifurcations arise as the value of B exceeds 3.44 and 3.56. This approach may help us to understand more about the patterning of the incidence of some diseases, particularly viral infections, which may exhibit a periodicity that can be explained by straightforward non-linear mathematics. Indeed disease patterns, population interventions and the attributes of a healthcare system may well interact in this non-linear manner, constituting complex and evolving systems in their own right (Tennison, 2002). At the root of this, in relation to the distinction between linear and non-linear systems, is the notion of *superposition*. In linear systems, the effect of the interaction of two variables, or two different causes, is merely the superposition of the combined effects of those two causes (Tennison, 2002). However, in a non-linear system, adding the effects of two elementary actions can lead to dramatic, unpredictable and novel properties, as a result of the co-operativity between the two actions or causes. It is this co-operativity or interaction that requires further research within the field of clinical medicine. How do we understand the co-operative interaction between two or more comorbid conditions? How much do we know about the interaction of medications for different conditions when taken in conjunction for decades? Given the description of complex systems presented here, and the evidence of their ubiquity, it is not unreasonable to consider the need to explore such questions from the non-linear perspective.

Complex responsive processes are a further useful notion within complexity which may be relevant in deepening our understanding of the interaction between doctor and patient during consultations. Remember Mrs B's consultation at the beginning of this book. This was one of a set of consultations, in this case going back a decade and a half, in which the participants – Mrs B and myself – were changed, both in relation to each other and in relation to the other systems (outside of the consultation in their own worlds) in which we participated. Nothing could have predicted the outcome of that consultation, although the conditions that led to it were all abundantly evidenced. My perception of the outcome was that it combined a more profound interpersonal relationship with this elderly woman, a greater respect for me (I sensed) on her part and, frankly, a poor therapeutic outcome in terms of a clinical plan. The greater trust that we both felt existed as a consequence of this event may in itself be seen as an emergent property of the series of interactions leading up to, and including, that consultation. Whatever conclusions one might reach, my argument is that the principles of complexity provide a fresh and, I assert, more valuable set of principles with which to explore and understand such consultations. In the next chapter I shall consider some examples which show how the principles of complexity have been deployed to address challenges in commerce, politics and healthcare, before setting out more formally some thoughts on a methodology that deploys those principles, with some examples of how they might be applied to clinical activities.

Chapter 6

Developing an understanding of chaos and complexity: implications and examples

Introduction

The aim of this book is to support the proposition that the explanatory model in contemporary medicine should be revised, and that this revision needs to accommodate a plurality of world-views. To this end, I have presented a conceptual exploration of the development and adequacy of medicine's contemporary explanatory model. This consisted of a review of the history of medicine, which showed how the model evolved and how science has come to occupy its hegemonic position. This model was then assessed in the light of two other intellectual traditions, namely the naturalistic and non-linear traditions, from which a number of observations can be made. I shall argue that there is a connection between an explanatory model, its epistemological framework and the tacit acceptance of a related world-view, or ontological perspective. Viewed in this way, it is argued that, in the practice of medicine, several ontological perspectives are deployed. Those that are explored in depth reflect a positivist reality (upon which the precepts of science are based), a socially constructed reality (from which the fruits of qualitative research have developed) and a relational reality (reflecting the dynamics of chaos and complexity). Each of these traditions can be pressed into service in medicine to help to make sense of the world from a particular point of view, by contributing through an expansion of human knowledge. Each tradition operates in a preferred domain.

Complementarity in world-views

The implications of the relationship between the three intellectual traditions described earlier are profound. Each has created a separate – but overlapping – explanatory model. Each explanatory model is the product of assumptions about reality (an ontology) and the way of knowing which makes sense of that world-view (an epistemology). This is how we each make sense of our world in our own way. We have a view of how the world works, and we devise ways of creating an understanding of it by developing types of knowledge that are compatible with that view, which help us to make sense of the world accordingly. Thus, as the outline of the three explanatory models described in this book implies, they are the product of different world-views – which are not mutually exclusive, but different. The scientific model is predicated on rational reductionism whose epistemology retains the notion of linearity, expressed as regular, proportionate and stable relationships between cause and effect. The naturalistic model accepts a more contextual, pluralist ontology in which a world-view is incrementally constructed through experience. The third view, based upon complexity, implies a world-view in which two principles, namely non-linearity and relational dynamics, are fundamental. The devices of its epistemological framework therefore populate that world-view and are compatible with it. The Stacey matrix, which is presented in a modified form in Figure 6.1, helps to explain the relationship between these traditions.

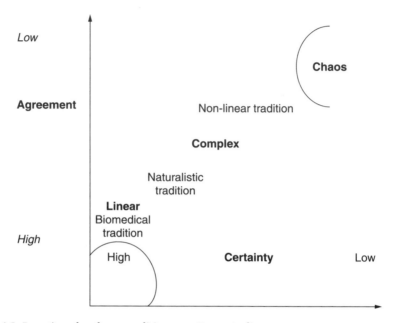

Figure 6.1 Locating the three traditions on Stacey's diagram.

The dominant explanatory model in medicine operates best where there is general agreement about the attributes of a system and a firm degree of certainty about the causal links between them. Such systems are mostly linear, so the explanatory model in medicine is seen operating best at or near the intersection of the two axes.

However, the characteristics of the naturalistic tradition allow it to flourish in less linear territory. Reflection upon the description by Smith and Heshusius (1986) of the relationship between quantitative and qualitative research in the latter part of the twentieth century suggests an evolving reciprocity or co-operation between these two approaches to investigation and knowledge. The naturalistic tradition can shed light on systems whose attributes are poorly understood, or on systems where the interactions between the components are less predictable and regular. The relationship between the two is reciprocal and can be cumulative. For example, we can describe the statistical benefits of warfarin in patients with atrial fibrillation and then, drawing on the naturalistic tradition, we can describe the struggle that doctors experience in implementing this scientifically robust piece of evidence.

The third tradition of non-linearity operates at the edge of chaos (Zimmerman and Plsek, 1998). Systems located in this space cannot be understood by applying a linear notion of cause and effect. They will develop self-organising behaviours, which will create emergent properties spontaneously, without a blueprint (Battram, 1998). Agents that participate in these systems develop the systems themselves, through co-creating processes of self-organisation (Wheatley, 2000). This is what distinguishes systems around this notional space from chaotic systems. Whereas the latter are the unpredictable outcome of the iterative application of deterministic mathematical formulae, the former can, through choice, change their rules of engagement and, as a consequence, the nature of their interaction. In terms of organisations, the progress of such systems cannot be managed by deploying command and control processes. Prediction is limited, and uncertainty is inherent. The distinction between linearity and non-linearity is not mutually exclusive – organisational systems can express themselves in both linear and non-linear terms. In the National Health Service, this is seen in hospitals that satisfy national targets by linearising their management approach (e.g. to meet mandatory Government targets) while deploying the principles of complexity (e.g. in transforming some of their services) (Plsek P, personal communication).

Implications

What then might be the implications of this relationship – this complementarity – between the three intellectual traditions described in the previous chapters? The implications can be considered both theoretically and practically.

Theoretical implications

The influence of the scientific approach to understanding the world, described in this book, has extended well beyond the fields in which it originated. Economics, sociology, politics and most recently international relations have all been heavily influenced by the scientific paradigm (Fukuyama, 1993). I have described how healthcare policy in the NHS has also been heavily influenced by a reductionist approach, expressed in the Taylorist predilection to view organisations as machines (Taylor, 1911). I argue, on the basis of the observations and evidence presented in this book, that healthcare policy should no longer predicate its policies on this reductionist, mechanical view of organisations. I have described a number of successful, explicit applications of an approach to organisational development and healthcare policy based on a clear understanding of complex adaptive systems (Zimmerman and Plsek, 1998; Plsek, 2000; Wheatley, 2000).

To this can be added the firm theory of the complexity of enabling infra-structures provided by Mitelton-Kelly (2003), which has progressed discussion about the relevance of complexity to organisational development (Durie *et al.*, 2004). Emphasising that complexity provides a conceptual framework for *thinking about* the world, as opposed to *seeing* the world, Mitelton-Kelly has reframed the principles of complexity for the context of organisational development. This reframing is summarised in Table 6.1. Although many of the implications and their consequences may be fairly familiar, Mitelton-Kelly's contribution has been to consolidate a theoretical basis for them.

The increasing acceptance of complexity in organisational research, both in the commercial world (Wheatley, 2000) and in the healthcare sector (Plsek, 2000;

Sweeney and Griffiths, 2002), will have implications for methods of research. At stake is the ability of research programmes to assist in contemporary sense making, as new complex and adapting systems evolve. In terms of data collection, this will afford a greater interest to storytelling and narrative analysis than before, and will rely more on experts on discourse and conversational analysis to apply their skills to analysing the co-creating conversations in healthcare (Snowden D, 2004, personal communication).

Table 6.1 Reframing the principles of complexity for organisations (Mitelton-Kelly, 2003)

Complexity principle	Application to organisational development
Complex responsive processes	The basic unit for the co-creation of a complex and adapting system. The outcomes of such conversations, in terms of actions or decisions, will ripple out and affect other parts of the system. Thus any 'improvement' arising in one part of the system may impose either 'benefit' or 'costs' on other related parts of the system
Relational dynamics	All the multiple dimensions of complex systems interact with each other. In human terms, this means that interpersonal, social, technical, economic and global dimensions may impinge upon and influence each other. Alterations in relational dynamics may change the rules of interaction. Agents that create such change do so by acting on limited local knowledge, not a comprehensive understanding of the whole system
Adaptation and co-evolution	The connectedness between individuals is not uniform, and it occurs both within and between systems. Individuals and their organisations exist in an ecosystem, in which adaptation by one part of the system alters the nature (fitness) of the system for other parts. Organisational thinking alters when one considers the possibilities of 'evolving with', rather than 'adapting to'. There is no hard boundary between a system and its environment
Self-organisation	The patterning of complex responsive processes can co-create relatively stable features of an organisation, as a result of adaptation and co-evolution. These structures cannot be predicted in advance, and do not develop as a result of a pre-ordained blueprint. The products of self-organising processes become the emergent properties of the system

Secondly, it should also endorse a layered approach to methodology. In this approach, initial qualitative and quantitative data are analysed for emerging themes (Creswell, 1988), and a second-level analysis from complexity is conducted on the themes that are identified. The report on the Pursuing Perfection Programme (a programme of transformational change in healthcare services in health and social care communities) described below serves as an example of this approach, and in the next chapter I shall illustrate this with some more examples from clinical research. Durie *et al.* (2004) have proposed a third-level analysis, incorporating workshops and exploring the implications for policy and practice, to complement the first two levels. The report on the Pursuing Perfection Programme is the first example of the application of such a method.

Practical applications of principles of complexity

A number of examples of the application of complexity principles to organisational change have already been cited (Zimmerman and Plsek, 1998; Wheatley, 2000). Three further examples of the application of complexity theory to transformational change are presented in this section, the first from the commercial world, and the other two demonstrating the relevance of complexity to national healthcare policy.

The European bank case study

Working with Papefthimiou, Mitelton-Kelly advised a large European bank on the reconfiguration of its entire information system, to prepare the organisation for the arrival of the new European currency – the euro (Mitelton-Kelly and Papefthimiou, 2000). The principles of complexity theory formed the basis for the advice that they gave and the research they conducted.

For the bank, the challenge was that the legal and regulatory frameworks for the introduction of the euro had been laid out, and their deadlines were clear. These arrangements constituted a necessary but in themselves insufficient set of conditions for change within the bank to occur. A raft of other conditions had to be created internally to establish a receptive framework, or enabling infrastructure, through which the bank could evolve broadly in a way that was consistent with achieving its goals. Prior to this change, the internal structure of the bank was such that systems developers, IT professionals, business managers and operations personnel rarely met each other, and as a result they simply did not talk to each other. Thus, although all of the agents in the system, namely the bank's employees, agreed on the nature of the goal (preparing the bank for the introduction of the euro), there was no effective enabling framework in place through which those agents could act together to achieve this goal.

The leadership necessary to facilitate coherent action around the agreed set of values (the bank had to maintain its reputation as it embraced the new currency regulations) was provided by the manager who oversaw the project. This manager:

- set up a programme of monthly meetings for all professional groups in the bank
- supported these meetings by providing weekly information updates for all personnel.

As a result of this:

- cross-dependencies between the participating groups were gradually identified (after a period of indifference to the programme itself)
- once these dependencies had been identified, new forms of communication emerged and new groups self-organised.

These processes and structures provided an enabling framework that was based on trust. Trust arose from the conversations, or complex responsive processes, whose patterning co-created the system's self-organisation, which is expressed in the new conditions for joint working. It grew out of the cross-dependencies, encouraged by the monthly meetings and weekly updates. From this perspective, trust became an emergent property of the system. In turn, the trust fed back, positively and iteratively, into the cross-dependencies, strengthening the conversations through which they were expressed. Sufficient continuity was ensured throughout the project by the monthly meetings, and the subsequent self-organisation of the professionals into autonomous groups, with the authority to experiment and take decisions within their domain of competence. Interestingly, the project manager introduced into the organisation an 'interpreter'– literally an agent who mediated dialogue between the domains of expertise that were represented at the meetings. However, the communications were never either managed or controlled from the top of the organisation.

The bank met its organisational goals in plenty of time for the introduction of the euro.

Pursuing Perfection Programme

The second completed study which supports the relevance of complexity theory to organisational change, this time in healthcare, describes the Pursuing Perfection Programme – a programme of transformational change in health and social care communities, which was conducted at four sites in the NHS in England (Sweeney, 2003b). In essence, four health and social care communities which had been selected to participate in this programme agreed to transform some services (initially two, then five more) around patients. The idea was to be radical, and to plan services around patients' lives, not the other way round (Bevan H, 2004, personal communication). From its inception, the programme was accompanied by a constructive enquiry, a process of research, which collated and commented upon the main themes constituting the programme's activities at each site. In summary, the enquiry consisted of a three-stage analysis. In the first stage, a standard case study was conducted (Creswell, 1988). In the second stage, the themes arising from this initial qualitative analysis were interrogated from the perspective of complexity (as in the case of the papers in Chapter 7). The third-level analysis took the form of workshops with fieldworkers, NHS professionals and organisational experts, at which the implications of the findings of the first two levels for policy and practice were debated. The methodology of this enquiry mirrors the second-level analysis of the empirical data presented in Chapter 7 of this book (Sweeney, 2003b).

The final report on this study, documenting the progress of two of the sites which succeeded in transforming their selected services, identified eight principal conditions which constituted the receptive context for whole-system transformational change within the participating organisations (Durie et al., 2004). These are shown in Table 6.2, where each of the conditions identified through the first-level analysis in the research on the Pursuing Perfection Programme is set out in the left-hand column, and the related feature of complex adaptive systems is shown in the right-hand column.

Table 6.2 The eight conditions that constitute the receptive context for whole-system transformational change (Durie *et al.*, 2004)

Condition for receptive context in the Pursuing Perfection Programme	Feature of complexity
Recognising that things are not working well enough, or could be done differently, with better outcomes for patients	Sensitivity to initial conditions. The necessary but in themselves insufficient conditions for change to occur
Leadership, demonstrating genuine commitment to aspirational goals. Visible behaviour change by leaders, indicating genuine commitment to the programme and to projects, with flexibility and comfort with ambiguity and emergence	Leadership to facilitate coherent action, as a prerequisite of an enabling framework
Behaviour change by the agents. Reconfiguration of relationships/creation of new relationships among staff, and between staff and patients	Reconfiguring relationships to co-create fresh complex responsive processes, whose patterning will help the system to self-organise
Encouraging a culture of experimentation and supported risk taking	Acceptance of inherent unpredictability in the system. Permission to allow interdependencies to coalesce into small self-organised experimenting groups
Accepting the possibility that different ways of working and thinking will be better for patients	The set of values which constitute receptive context
Genuine and meaningful patient involvement	The set of values that constitute receptive context
The importance of language (including the challenge of professional language) and communication (between and within organisations)	The importance of communication as the bedrock of the complex responsive processes whose patterning co-creates coherent behaviours and outcomes
Pursuing Perfection as a 'Way of Working'	The emergent property of coherent action. Not just 'another project', but a new way of working

There are similarities between the themes in this study of the Pursuing Perfection Programme and the study by Mitelton-Kelly and Papefthimiou (2000). Both accepted the external environment as a necessary but insufficient condition for change, both identified the need for new relationships (achieved by the monthly meetings in the European bank case study and by the reconfiguration of relationships in the Pursuing Perfection Programme) as a way of co-creating new complex responsive processes, and both recognised a set of values as the 'glue' for holding the emerging behaviour of the system together. The culture of experimentation that was fostered in the Pursuing Perfection Programme and the trust that was engendered in the European bank case study constitute the respective emergent properties of the system.

A strategy for containing AIDS: the experience of Brazil

The third example of the application of complexity theory to healthcare policy describes the Brazilian government's strategy to contain the AIDS epidemic in Brazil.

In the 1980s, Brazil had one of the highest infection rates for AIDS in the world (Darlington, 2000). With an accelerating infection rate for the virus far in excess of that in South Africa, coupled with an annual per capita income of less than $5000, the World Bank predicted disaster, calculating that Brazil would have 1.2 million cases of AIDS by 2000 (World Bank, 1997). In fact, in that year 0.5 million cases were reported to the World Health Organization, representing an infection rate of 0.6%, compared with a rate of 25% in South Africa (World Health Organization, 2002).

Gloubermann and Zimmerman's (2002) careful analysis of the World Bank's appraisal reveals how the Bank's predictions were predicated on a linear modelling of the issues. This led them to develop complicated rather than complex assumptions about Brazil's predicament, from which an apocalyptic picture emerged, predicting disaster for the country. The World Bank's assumptions included the following.

- Effective treatment, in the form of antiretroviral treatment, is too demanding of clinical services in poor developing countries.
- Poor countries rapidly realise that they cannot sustain the cost of effective treatments, so they concentrate exclusively on prevention.
- Even if drug treatment is available for some AIDS patients, the ill-educated, barely literate people, who are typical of the AIDS patients in poor countries, cannot possibly manage their own complicated drug regimes.
- The way to implement effective prevention is to scare people – fear of death will limit the spread of the disease.
- Effective prevention still results in huge losses to the current adult generation, and its benefits will take two or three generations to accrue.
- An integrated programme of prevention and treatment in combination is beyond the organisational capacity of poor and developing countries.

Analysing the Brazilian authorities' approach to this challenge, the authors describe what happened, before examining those actions from the perspective of complexity. The Brazilian government's actions included the following.

- They gave the drugs away free. They took a risky decision to manufacture their own generic brands of the antiretroviral preparations, which up to that time had been produced expensively, mostly in the USA, by huge international pharmaceutical companies. The risk lay in a legal stand-off with the pharmaceutical giants, who after nearly two years decided not to pursue the government for breach of patent. By 2000, eight of the 12 available preparations were produced generically in Brazil, and consequently the costs of treatment turned out to be between 65% and 90% less expensive than in the USA, upon whose figures the World Bank had based their calculations.
- They used treatment as a part of the prevention strategy, figuring that, when people know that they will receive free treatment, they will be more willing to attend for therapy. Those patients who did so received preventive advice, spread

the word to the close communities in which the disease was rife, and felt their decisions reinforced as the progression of their symptoms slowed down.

- The Brazilian authorities accepted poor literacy and numeracy in their target population as a challenge, and developed a huge number of creative ways of tackling it. Doctors and nurses co-opted other healthcare workers, lay people and patients themselves to produce their own ideas of how to get the key messages across. Drawings of food were used to remind people when to take the pills. Arrangements were made for food to be provided free through schools and churches, giving a further point for compliance messages to be reinforced. Humour became a key ingredient of billboards advertising free condoms.
- The Brazilian government seized upon the AIDS epidemic as an opportunity to strengthen its healthcare infrastructure, rather than simply seeing it as the reason for their failure to control the problem. They deployed over 600 pre-existing non-governmental and community organisations to access hard-to-reach groups, and they established a network of over 130 testing and counselling centres (Centre for Disease Control, 2000).

From the perspective of complexity, what the Brazilian government did was to accept and make use of the messiness in their healthcare system, by maximising the connectivity of the existing informal, social and community relationships. They knew that they had a receptive context – a focus on potentially shared activities (the care of AIDS patients), which all constituents agreed was mainstream business (no one was in any doubt about the fact that the country faced a catastrophe). By facing up to the pharmaceutical giants, the Brazilian government exhibited sufficient leadership to facilitate the interaction of the other agents in the system. As a result, the system self-organised – with AIDS patients redefining their informal groups as patient groups receiving treatment and preventive advice. And the system co-evolved – churches and other non-governmental organisations became actively involved as agents of the healthcare system. Positive feedback, in the form of descriptions of symptomatic improvement by AIDS patients themselves, reinforced the self-organising processes and supported the emergent approach taken by the authorities.

In summary, as Gloubermann and Zimmerman (2002) have expressed it, they reframed complicated questions as complex challenges. When the World Bank had asked 'Who can you afford to treat? What will you have to cut back on to afford this?' – linear questions – the Brazilian government asked 'How can we reduce the cost of treatment so that we can provide it for everyone?' – a question that demands a non-linear, emergent solution. 'What infrastructure do you need? And from what existing service will you take the money to pay for it?', the World Bank asked. The Brazilians transformed this into the following questions: 'Where and what are the pre-existing informal arrangements that we can deploy as part of an emerging infrastructure and how can we strengthen them?'. Complicated became complex, predetermined became emergent, and a shortage of resource was redefined as potential abundance.

Implications for practice: epidemiology and public health

The distinction between chaos and complexity explains why early research into the implications of non-linear systems for clinical medicine focused on the relevance of chaotic mathematical modelling to clinical issues. Where systems can be described numerically, sometimes with great precision, their iterative patterning becomes a real possibility, holding out the potential to elicit features of chaotic systems, such as period doubling or bifurcation. A number of the examples from clinical medicine illustrate this point.

One of the first examples of this was an important paper by Schaffer (1985) that modelled the spread of infectious disease using simultaneous non-linear equations. Although the mathematics in Schaffer's paper are beyond the non-specialist, the author presents a complete non-linear mathematical modelling of infectious disease spread, showing that it exhibits fractal patterning and has a positive Lyapunov exponent, which shows sensitivity to initial conditions (*see* Chapter 7), both of which are essential features of chaotic systems.

Here Schaffer is exploiting the analogy between the biological species modelling described in Chapter 7 and the infectious agent process. More recently, Tennison (2002) has shown how the non-linear equation used to model species survival can, with sufficient simplifications, be applied to the spread of infectious diseases. Thus the equation becomes:

$$X_{t+1} = a_{xt} (1 - x_t)$$

where t denotes time, x denotes the point prevalence of the disease at time t, and a denotes the virulence of the infecting agent, which is a variable, not a constant, and can change over time. Such variation may, for example, be due to climate change, genetic drift or the effect of other organisms. Iterative solving of this equation, for variable values of a, produces the same bifurcations and period doubling as were discussed on p. 68 in relation to species survival. But how does this help public health specialists? Epidemiologists have long been familiar with the cyclical patterns of incidence of certain viral infections, including measles and pertussis. They are also familiar with diseases such as psittacosis and plague, whose incidence seems to be quite random, and they recognise that yet other diseases, such as multiple sclerosis, exhibit long-term trends (called secular trends) for no obvious reason. The value of non-linear modelling, and the attendant possibilities of period doubling (sometimes with long period intervals), allow epidemiologists to speculate that these diseases might have an underlying dynamic, with an oscillation in infectivity over long time periods, similar to the period-doubling models of species survival. Speculating about the potential of non-linear modelling in infectious epidemiology, Tennison (2002) acknowledges that 'even a highly simplified non-linear model exhibits remarkably complicated behaviour, similar to that seen in the real world.' Some parts of complexity theory, Tennison concludes, have great potential relevance for epidemiology – for example, in the more accurate planning of vaccination campaigns.

Example: cardiology

Cardiology provides an example of the potential of chaos and complexity theory to lead to a revision of basic assumptions about the underlying conventional models. Bifurcation is now a well-studied phenomenon in cardiology, and Goldberger and West (1987) have contributed to an understanding of period doubling in sick sinus syndrome. Fractal patterning (the tendency for self-similarity within the period-doubling trends in chaotic systems) occurs at the

His–Purkinje conduction network. Healthy heart rate variability has also been shown to have a fractal structure, the loss of which appears to be associated with a poor prognosis, suggesting that chaos underpins normal cardiac function. In their review of the applications of non-linear dynamics to clinical cardiology (Goldberger and West, 1987), the authors speculate about fractal patterning (they use the term 'fractal anatomy') in the pulmonary, hepato-biliary and renal systems.

Example: diabetes

In diabetes, the degree to which chaos and complexity have been applied is less advanced than in cardiology or epidemiology, but non-linear models have been suggested, and considerable speculation now underpins the debate about optimising diabetes management, drawing on non-linear mathematics. Holt (2002a) disputes the conventional biomedical explanation of diabetes as a state of relative or absolute insulin deficiency, with or without insulin resistance, arguing that any predictive modelling for a patient with diabetes that is based upon linear thinking has the ability to predict fluctuations in blood sugar levels for a period of only 15 days (Liska-Hackzell, 1999). This analysis raises serious questions about the routine staging of appointments at diabetic clinics at the current 3-monthly intervals.

Holt (2002a) presents the conventional understanding of blood glucose behaviour as:

$$G(\text{postprandial}) = G(\text{preprandial}) + a(C - I)$$

where C is the amount of carbohydrate eaten at the last meal, and I is the amount of insulin injected or secreted since. Conventionally, 'a' is taken to be a constant that is determined by patient-specific parameters such as body mass index or insulin sensitivity. This has given rise to a negative feedback, equilibrium-based model of diabetes in which, so long as C 'balances' I at each meal, the blood glucose behaviour will remain stable. However, as Baxt (1994) pointed out 10 years ago, it has been a common misconception in pathophysiology generally to mistake a variable for a constant, and it is Holt's contention that 'a' in the above equation is better understood as a variable, in which case the equation becomes non-linear. The additional features which contribute to 'a' and render it variable include the impaired ability of the system (that is, the diabetic patient) to detect movements of glucose levels away from normal, the inability to respond to such swings when they occur, and the presence of positive feedback. The source of the positive feedback consists of the behavioural mechanisms that affect some patients with diabetes, which tend to move the system further away from normal – for example, inactivity, lethargy, and inaccurate or missed insulin dosage. Further positive feedback, in the longer term, comes from the cycle of increased insulin levels leading to weight gain, which leads to an increased insulin dose, and so on. Holt is careful to state 'some' patients, as others can sense these fluctuations and react appropriately, suggesting that there is a balance between negative and positive feedback, which is likely to vary between individuals. Drawing upon the insights from the work of Garfinkel *et al.* (1992) in cardiology, Holt speculates about the potential for a non-linear adaptive algorithm to help patients with diabetes to manage fluctuations in blood sugar levels. Any such adaptive algorithm, Holt suggests, would require attention to the behavioural characteristics of the individual, reflecting the contribution of positive feedback within the system, and awareness of blood glucose levels without testing (to enable reaction to small perturbations), and residual endogenous insulin secretion, the presence of which might allow the system to settle at a displaced stable position, say with a slightly higher 'normal' stable range of blood sugar concentration. Although as yet there is no firm empirical basis for confirming or refuting Holt's speculation, the author commends the use of prolonged one-dimensional time-series data, plotting blood sugar level at time 'G_t', and against blood sugar level one time interval later at 'G_{t+1}', and repeating this over many hundred data points, on the grounds that chaotic systems can sometimes be revealed in this way (Rossler and Rossler, 1994).

Implications for research

Researching health technology as a complex system

Support for the analytical approach (Sweeney, 2003b; Durie *et al.*, 2004) and applied to the empirical data is found in Griffiths' description (2002) of the methodology in her research on the impact of new technologies. In the course of this research, Griffiths explored in detail the impact of two new technologies, namely mammography and bone densitometry, on middle-aged women.

Griffiths argues at the outset that her subject matter can only be explored by seeing it as a complex system, in this case bounded by the policy, practice and consequences of technological innovation. The impact of such technology is predicated on complex responsive processes and characterised by iteration, feedback and co-evolution. In her research she adopts a dual approach, termed 'fine and coarse grain', to her exploration of the impact of new technology, acknowledging that health technologies are shaped by society and that they in turn shape society. Further interactions and feedback within the system become the focus for the research's interest at three levels:

1 those developing and providing the technology
2 those using the products of their innovation
3 those observing and commenting on it publicly (government reports) and privately (e.g. carers and colleagues of users).

At the 'fine-grain' level of research, Griffiths and her colleagues focus on the interactions between those providing new technologies (in this case mammography and bone densitometry) and those consuming them (middle-aged women). These can be seen as the complex responsive processes that co-create the impact of the technology. Data at this level are collated from descriptive quantitative data (what is being used?) and detailed qualitative data (how is it being used?). At the 'coarse-grain' level, the focus becomes the macro-issues, such as the cultural, policy and organisational issues at regional or national level that form the system's (loose) boundaries. Material from this level of research is drawn from government reports, professional guidelines, guides from self-help or voluntary groups, or commentaries in the media. This level of the research accepts that the environment in which the technology is provided will impact on, and in turn be affected by, the experience of providers and users. The researchers look for patterns in their data – patterns of response, use, comment and user experience – which constitute the system's emergent properties (Griffiths, 2002). Their search for patterning parallels the second-level analysis of the empirical data described in Chapter 7. Griffiths adopts a co-evolutionary approach to her material, assuming that change is occurring in all of the interacting populations of the system under scrutiny, and accepting that, as a consequence, change can be driven in both directions by both positive and negative feedback, and between the participants at the 'coarse' and 'fine' levels of activity.

The research described here, together with the example from Durie *et al.* (2004) described earlier, has implications for this type of health services research generally. Henceforth, research methods will benefit from considering both the linear and non-linear features of any domain. In clinical research it will always be necessary to explore as robustly as possible the basic science of a problem, its pathophysiology and any proposed technical intervention (the linear side of the domain). What we learn from complexity is that this is not enough. The subsequent interaction, between innovators, developers, providers, users and their carers, needs to be rigorously described in order to capture the reality of a system in which use (or disuse) of an innovation is accepted as an emergent property of the system, co-created by the complex responsive processes of its agents (technicians, guideline developers, patients and carers). This aspect of health-related research will combine both conventional quantitative data and methods (how much of this innovation is being used?) and qualitative data and methods (how is this being done?), looking for patterns within the data which represent iterative feedback and co-evolution within the system that is under scrutiny.

Implications for healthcare policy

The ubiquity of complex systems seriously calls into question the rationale behind command and control management policy in healthcare. Identifying what they call co-evolutionary dynamics, Volberda and Lewin (2003) call on policy makers to commit themselves rather to guiding the evolution of behaviours that emerge in the course of the interaction of independent agents within any system. Policy makers, these authors argue, need to encourage self-organisation, recognising the potential of organisations always – through the patterning of their complex responses – to find order, however complex or convoluted the environment. Healthcare research needs to take account of co-evolution, focusing on the emergent properties of a system (that is, a healthcare organisation or community). These emergent properties arise from the micro-state adaptations that are co-created by the system's internal complex responsive processes, and the macro-state adaptations that reflect the community's interaction with the wider environment. The authors' recommendation for the more widespread use of longitudinal time-series data sets has implications for the funding of health-related research. If one cannot predict either how long it will take for a system to evolve, or what direction that evolution might take, how can one frame research projects that are 'good enough'? One response, currently supported by the Modernisation Agency of the Department of Health, and applied to the Pursuing Perfection Programme in the NHS in the UK, is to undertake policy innovation and research concurrently, speculating initially about how much time will be 'enough', before gradually building up experience of just how much time is likely to be needed to make intelligent observations.

Summary

We are now in a position to restate the key themes in the debate about explanatory models, and their relationship to ways of knowing. This book asserts that the conventional explanatory model in biomedicine is predicated on scientific positivism but that, in practice, professionals deploy a range of 'ways of knowing' which take advantage of appropriate features of the three traditions described in the preceding chapters, pressing them into service where appropriate. My contention is that practitioners do this tacitly and subconsciously. However, when the features of and relationship between the three traditions are set out, one is forced to consider more explicitly the relationship between ways of knowing and the nature of clinical practice. Mrs B's consultation illustrated the tension that is created when two traditions clash. In these situations, one is compelled to ask which tradition should predominate. How do we judge when best to deploy one way of knowing against another? And who decides this? The centrality of complex responsive processes to the interaction between doctor and patient, and the subtlety of the inexorable changes that emerge from such iterative interactions, compel practitioners to focus very precisely on a number of issues. These include the way we explain things, the reciprocity of the doctor–patient–doctor relationship (which is mutually changing, not the one-way traffic suggested, for example, by the term 'compliance'), and the way we as practitioners change as a consequence of our interaction with a whole range of patients – as well as our interaction with the other systems in which we participate. From Chapter 5, it is clear that the other sciences have accepted the challenge of modifying their explanatory models as a result of their learning about the principles of chaos and complexity. We await such a response from the biomedical community, where the algorithmic bastions of explanation remain unbreached. However, before considering the future, I want to develop some ideas about the implications of complexity for research in medicine, by considering – from the perspective of complexity – some examples of a second-level analysis of data that were collected during four standard research projects conducted in primary care. The purpose of the next chapter is to demonstrate the practical applications of complexity principles to the contexts described in the examples that are presented.

Chapter 7

Using complexity principles in healthcare research: examples of data analysis using complexity principles

Introduction

This chapter presents four original papers, published in peer-reviewed journals in the fields of health and social care, which show how the principles of complexity can be incorporated into a research methodology in order to deepen our understanding of some common challenges in general practice. Each of the papers is reproduced in full, as published, in the Appendix, and a short résumé is presented here.

Thus the aims of this chapter are as follows:

- to present empirical data which develop the conceptual exploration of the adequacy of the explanatory model in contemporary medicine
- to interrogate the main themes in four empirical papers from the perspective of complex adaptive systems
- to identify any emerging hypotheses suggested by this analysis
- to commend possible avenues of future research based on the foregoing.

Four papers (in all of which the author was involved) are presented. In each case a short résumé is set out, to which are added some reflections on the research projects, enabled by re-presenting some of the original data which were omitted due to the editorial constraints of the journals in which the papers appeared. I hope that by introducing this additional original data, the second-level analysis, drawing on the principles of complexity, will be made clearer.

The methodology: second-level analysis from complexity

The methodology used in this analysis has been developed and deployed successfully in research that I have conducted with the Health Complexity Group of the Peninsula Medical School of the Universities of Exeter and Plymouth. The method has been described theoretically (Sweeney, 2003b), and was implemented recently in a national study of transformational change in NHS health and social care communities (Durie *et al.*, 2004). In principle, this approach involves a detailed mixed qualitative and quantitative case study at its first level. At the second level, the themes identified via the first-level analysis are explored for any insight which either confirms or disputes key features of complex systems. These features, which were explained in Chapter 5, are as follows:

- receptive context (an enabling framework or infrastructure of communicability conducive to an agreed purpose)
- complex responsive processes (the conversations which constitute the primary unit of a complex adaptive system involving people, through which they co-create the system)
- self-organisation (the evolution of coherent units or behaviours consistent with that purpose)
- co-evolution (identified through sustained and adaptive patterns of behaviours consistent with the overall purpose)
- emergence (the unifying feature, an epi-phenomenon created by the patterning of interaction of a system's agents).

Great care is exercised at the second level not to 'read into' the data possible connections with complexity. The aim is to reflect on the data as they stand, drawing on the principles of complexity, to determine the value of any insights (from that perspective) for transferability and learning. Should the themes identified in the four papers in this chapter not yield any insights consistent with the features of complex systems, this would be revealed and discussed.

The criteria for identifying the presence of a receptive context are set out in Chapters 5 and 6. Thus the absence of a receptive context is taken as sufficient grounds for assuming that the system under scrutiny was not complex. The presence of a receptive context, coupled with evidence of self-organisation through the patterning of complex responsive processes, is accepted as the minimum condition under which it becomes justifiable to describe the system under scrutiny as complex. In the papers analysed in this chapter, these criteria were applied after the data had been collected and had undergone first-level qualitative analysis.

Paper 1

Evidence-based practice: can this help joint working?
Published in 2000 in *Managing Community Care*. **8**: 21–7.

Background

The first paper captures the findings of a small qualitative study which compared the way in which participating health and social care professionals conceptualised the medical model, in its contemporary form of evidence-based medicine, and how they compared that with what they called the social model. The paper capitalised on a rare opportunity in which a range of health and social care professionals had come together for a study day to learn about and discuss evidence-based medicine. The purpose of the study day was to provide a workshop introducing the basic principles of critical appraisal, and to explore, in small group work, the participants' attitudes to and beliefs about evidence-based medicine. The study day took place against a backdrop of little evidence, within that health and social care community, of joint working in the context of evidence-based practice.

Method

This was a small opportunistic study comprising three focus groups consisting of a mixture of health and social care professionals. The health professionals were drawn from primary care, and included general practitioners and practice and district nurses, as well as representatives of the professions allied to medicine. A grounded theory approach to data analysis was adopted (Creswell, 1988).

Main results

Two main themes emerged. These related to views on evidence-based practice, and perceived barriers to working together. Under the latter theme, three sub-themes were identified, namely operational matters, the metaphysics of health-care, and philosophical differences in the conceptual modelling of health and social care.

The participants said that the prospect of health and social care professionals working together more closely was welcomed, and that evidence-based practice should be encouraged and financially supported. There were difficulties in applying evidence derived from population studies to individuals, and also in applying evidence from a study undertaken in a locality that may be quite different from the participants' home territory. Evidence-based practice might also present a threat. For example, one healthcare professional remarked, 'Do I really want to accept I've been doing something futile for 20 years?'.

Although the participants regarded joint working positively, they bemoaned the difficulties of getting 'the right people round the table.' All three groups agreed that the public's rising expectations of health and social care services, and their increasing demands, were stressful. In addition, patients presented not with discreetly packaged issues, but with undifferentiated problems whose origin lay to a large extent in their unique personal and social circumstances.

Two of the groups identified serious conceptual difficulties in working together, based on a perceived dichotomy of approach between health and social care: 'The basis of the assessment is different – GPs think in terms of treatment' and 'We've got the problem of them working most specifically with the social model as opposed to the medical model.'

All three groups explored perceived differences between the medical and social models of practice. The data are best illustrated by the following extract: 'Medicine is much more easily definable . . . with medication you either take it or you don't; with social services you are talking about people and there are an infinite variety of variables.' This perceived difference in professional approach extended not only to the assessment of individual cases, but also to the application of research evidence, and to treatment decisions generally.

Conclusion

There is both a general willingness among these health and social care professionals to work together, and enthusiasm for evidence-based practice. Factors over and above the research evidence have an impact on the willingness of the groups to work together. These include metaphysical factors, by which is meant the personal unhappiness or insuperable disadvantage of some patients. Distinct differences existed in the ways in which each of the two groups (health and social care) conceptualised the other's discipline.

Commentary on Joint Working Paper

This is clearly a small and opportunistic study, and as such its findings must be viewed as a snapshot of how a mixed group of health and social care professionals express their views about the nature of their professional practice, rather than anything more definitive. On the other hand, it is extremely unusual for such diverse groups to come together for such a discussion – sufficiently rare for the editor of this respected peer-reviewed journal of social care to be anxious to present the findings. It seemed to be too good an opportunity to miss.

The main concern about the publication of this paper was the shortage of editorial space afforded by the editor. Clearly this constrained the way in which we could present our data and methods. It also had the effect of abbreviating some of the results sections in a way that reduced the impact of three key themes. These were to do with context, and with what we called the metaphysical and philosophical levels of interpretation. In order to gain a clearer understanding of how a second-level analysis from complexity might proceed, I have gone back to the original data, to expand on these themes, before commenting on their relevance.

Context

The original data set contained a separate category entitled 'geography'. This category contained participants' comments on their own locality – that is, the physical context in which they operated. The importance of this category lay in the way in which the participants appeared to be saying that *where* they worked affected *how* they worked. As such this seemed to be significant, as it limited the way in which they approached the whole notion of applying the scientific method (in the shape of evidence-based medicine) to their routine working practice. In the final draft only six lines were retained by the editor in this area. The following paragraph re-presents the relevant original data under this category.

The groups spent some time describing how their own working practice was affected by the specific geographical characteristics of their localities. For example, one seaside town appeared to be 'detached' or 'peripheral' and 'very rural and spread out'. Poor transport connections were blamed for creating this 'out here' feeling. Demography also had an effect on working practice. These localities had a high rate of unemployment that was weakened by a seasonal influx of a population seeking part-time work. This seasonal influx was not wholly welcomed for other reasons: 'the influx of some of our visitors leads to drug and alcohol problems'. One participant summed up these themes as follows: 'A lot of the links we have to make tend to be in [name of town], a lot of resources are centralised – that actually is quite a barrier when it comes to working at a local level.' Thus described, the locality context appeared to have an impact not simply on participants' own work, but also on their enthusiasm for working together.

Metaphysical level

Although this heading was retained by the editor, the final paper omitted what seemed, from the poignancy of the data, to be an important reference to the very private view participants held about the nature of their own work, and the way in which working models, which gave rise to their professional boundaries, appeared at times to be confusing. The following extract presents the original data in this area:

> *A set of data was identified under the broad heading of working together which seemed to transcend mere day-to-day operational issues and dwelt upon the inherent nature of the problems faced by these professional groups which in itself might render joint working difficult. Some of these were generic. 'We all carry a fantasy of what's going on in our heads', observed one participant. Another felt the fact that 'we are all faced with personal unhappiness and distress' could be dispiriting and as a result dampen enthusiasm for col-laboration. The group also recognised that professional demarcation, in terms of responsibility, did not always appear sensible: a dichotomy of medical versus social model emerged. 'Take baths, for example: is this a medical or social bath?'*

Philosophical level

Although the final paper retained almost all of the original interpretation of the participants' data, the following section highlights the consistency of this theme of perceived difference in the approach to assessing patients held by these groups of combined health and social care professionals:

> *This perceived difference in professional approach extended not only to the assessment of individual cases but to treatment decisions generally and to the application of research evidence. 'It would be interesting to see, working with the social model or the medical model, what those differences are.' One participant argued that the medical model takes away responsibility, 'you know using the medical evidence of the clinical diagnosis', while the social model was characterised 'by working with the person.' Judging by the amount of data collected under this heading, this theme was seen as central.*

Summary of Joint Working Paper

Two main observations can be made from this small study. First, given the opportunity, these health and social care professionals were able to express profound views about the nature of their responsibility, which went beyond the simple application of clinical evidence to reflect on the impact of metaphysics – patients' unhappiness, suffering and despair – on their enthusiasm for working together. Secondly, they held contrasting views about the nature of medical and social care, and they framed this comparison with fairly adversarial metaphors – 'the problem' or 'polarisation'.

Paper 2

A preliminary study of the decision-making process within general practice
Published in 2000 in *Family Practice*. 17: 428–9.

Background

This study sought to establish an empirical basis for the notion of personal significance, described in Chapter 3, by exploring the factors that contribute to the process of decision making within general practice, over and above evidence-based information. Awareness of the latest scientific evidence, as well as the ability to critically appraise literature and assess its generalisability, have been identified as integral to the practice of evidence-based medicine. However, the evaluation of evidence in general practice is often illogical and irrational (Sweeney, 1996), and it cannot be assumed that GPs practise the principles underpinning evidence-based medicine in their decision making.

Method

A qualitative study was conducted using semi-structured interviews on a purposive sample of five GPs, based in south-west England. Each interview was tape-recorded and transcribed verbatim.

Main results

Six themes emerged from the data, namely practitioner, patient, practitioner–patient relationship, verbal and non-verbal communication, evidence-based medicine and external factors. These are addressed in sequence.

All of the practitioners described how previous clinical experiences and their own clinical beliefs had an impact on clinical decision making: 'doctors also have their own philosophy of health' (Interview 1) and 'it's the things that go wrong that imprint on your memory . . .' (Interview 3). Equally, the participants recognised that understanding patients' cultural beliefs, background and attitudes is integral to the decision-making process. One general practitioner remarked 'You have to know where the patients are coming from . . . and what their beliefs are' (Interview 1). These two features constituted the bedrock of the practitioner–patient relationship, which the participants described as constantly evolving, and for the sake of which the practitioners were at times able to bow to the patient's expectations for the sake of maintaining good relations: 'the nature of the relationship is one that continues and goes on and there may be far more important issues coming up than this trivial issue of whether or not you prescribe penicillin . . .' (Interview 1).

To develop the relationship, the practitioners acknowledged the importance of communication, not only in terms of their own language – 'you've got to pitch what you say at a level that the patient will understand . . .' (Interview 3) – but also by sensitively observing sensitive cues from patients – 'patients do give quite strong messages, without necessarily expressing them verbally, about what they want' (Interview 1). As far as evidence-based medicine was concerned, the participating doctors accepted its contribution in a qualified way: 'EBM measures the things that can be measured . . .' (Interview 2). However, external factors influenced the decision-making process as well: 'GPs are conscious of society's views, but particularly cost' (Interview 3), 'time is critical, we don't have very long, that's the problem' (Interview 5) and 'the media are more powerful than anything else' (Interview 5).

Conclusion

Consideration needs to be given to the way in which the nature of the decision-making process impacts on the way that 'evidence' is constructed and promoted in general practice.

Commentary on the preliminary study of the decision-making process within general practice

As its title suggests, this was a preliminary study, and its results and contribution should be considered alongside the next paper in this chapter (Freeman and Sweeney, 2001). The enquiry was sparked off by a discussion with the co-author about the meaning of the term 'linear' when applied to explanatory models. Evidence-based medicine had been criticised for being algorithmic. There was, it had been argued, a linear sequence in its five-stage approach. But was this, we thought, the way it actually happened in practice? How did decisions evolve within consultations? If evidence-based medicine was linear, this assumed the existence of an opposite, non-linear approach. What, then, might be the attributes of such a non-linear system? This was the discussion which provided the impetus for this small study.

Comments on the data

As the editor of the journal in which this paper was published presented it as a short report, much of the original data, as well as clarification of the methods, was excluded. As the themes in this short study are relevant to the argument, I have gone back to the original data to report them in greater depth. The headings that were used in the published paper have been retained.

Practitioner

When using the phrase 'philosophy of health', the practitioners in this study appeared to mean their own values – 'you make value judgments all the time' (Interview 5) – and this sometimes conflicted with professionals' values. One practitioner said 'I'm not quite sure where to draw the line between what I believe in and what is acceptable as a GP' (Interview 2). Several participants stressed the importance of previous clinical experiences as an influence on the way in which they consulted: 'If you've had a patient who has a problem, and dies from a stroke, a bleed due to warfarin, then you're going to be cagey about putting other people on to it' (Interview 4).

Patient

The implications of accommodating the patient's health beliefs, referred to in the published text, were spelled out in several interviews. 'The evidence is always tempered by the patient and the doctor,' reflected one general practitioner, 'but particularly by the patient' (Interview 3). Sometimes this might mean that robust research evidence would be ignored 'if the patients don't believe it works' (Interview 3). Another practitioner summed up the tension as follows: 'The evidence is cold and we are about managing patients' (Interview 1).

Practitioner–patient relationship

The use of the word 'Technicolor' to describe the doctor's relationship with a patient is intriguing, and suggests an entity that is rich, multi-faceted and difficult to quantify. 'There is some logic in it,' one GP said, 'but you certainly can't quantify it and write it down in a flow diagram' (Interview 2).

Verbal and non-verbal communication

In addition to recognising the importance of semantics in conveying important messages – and receiving verbal clues from patients – referred to in the published text, the general practitioners stressed the importance of reciprocity in these consultations by adding, for example, that 'You can make a remark or a question which shows that you're on line, then you're away . . . similarly if you ask a question which shows you're not, they'll stay dumb and blocked' (Interview 4). Patients pick up on doctors' 'styles' (Interview 4) and, as one doctor admitted, they can 'select themselves out and shop around . . . I do appreciate that there are more patients who are not suitable for my approach than are suitable' (Interview 4).

Evidence-based medicine

A perceived advantage of evidence-based medicine for the doctors in this study was that it provided a yardstick to use when coming to an agreement about when a new piece of evidence should change their own, and their partnership's, practice: 'we would normally need something of the level of . . . um . . . a *BMJ* article or *Lancet* editorial' (Interview 3). In several interviews, the doctors at this point often reflected on the tension between clinical significance and personal significance. One doctor commented about patients who might say: 'Oh, he's taken me off my X drug which I've been perfectly happy with . . .' to a new (evidence-based drug) which 'provokes anxiety and people feel nervous about it . . . saying look at all these side-effects' (Interview 1). An interesting distinction was made by one doctor between vigorously treating risk factors and relieving suffering: 'when somebody is having a clear-cut piece of suffering which we're trying to relieve and the further away we get from that the harder it is to fit the evidence with a person and a practical situation' (Interview 4).

Summary

The central observation from this study relates to the importance of the evolving relationships that doctors elaborate with their patients, and vice versa (as we are reminded by one participant in this study). This idea of two people contributing to and being mutually influenced by their evolving relationship echoes the definition of complex responsive processes that was developed in Chapter 5. I shall return to this later, in the second-level analysis of all four papers in the final section of this chapter.

Paper 3

Why general practitioners do not implement evidence: a qualitative study
Published in 2001 in *BMJ*. **323**: 1100–14.

Background

This paper extends the line of enquiry that was initiated in the previous paper by exploring, through the medium of Balint groups, the reasons why general practitioners do not always implement best evidence. The aim was to supplement the empirical basis supporting the relevance of personal significance to clinical practice, by reflecting on how doctors crafted their decisions during consultations.

Method

A total of 19 general practitioners took part in 13 Balint group meetings, for 11 of which data were available for analysis.

Main results

The process of implementing clinical evidence is affected by the personal and professional experiences of the doctor. For example, one participant remarked that: 'I actually had two 50-year-olds who had strokes from atrial fibrillation because they didn't get warfarin . . . that really hit me.' Others described how, having initially been less than enthusiastic about anticoagulating patients with atrial fibrillation, subsequent positive clinical experience could change their view – 'I'm back on it.' The main point of this theme is expressed thus: 'We are influenced at least as much, if not more, by the experiences of individual patients as we are by the evidence.' This suggests that the relationship that the doctor has with individual patients also affects the process of implementing evidence, a second strong theme that emerged from the data. 'Even if the evidence was extremely good,' one general practitioner said, 'most of us would only ever interpret it in the context of the patient.' This was not a one-way process, and patients could, at times, and as a function of their relationship with the doctor, influence the doctor's decisions. This is summed up by the following quote: 'Well, he's a farmer, so every time he calls the vet he gets antibiotics.'

When describing the clinical applications of evidence-based medicine, these participants depicted a tension between primary and secondary care. The doctors thought that specialists approach evidence-based practice differently. For example, they do not realise how tricky it is to control some common conditions. 'You get stroppy letters from the clinic saying your patient's blood pressure is still 160,' said one participant, 'and I go . . . yes, yes, I know. You feel under pressure from the guidelines, but you know it's not for want of trying.'

In addition, the practitioner's feelings – not just about their relationships with patients, but also about the evidence itself – modify the way in which clinical evidence is applied. The very presence of 'evidence' – for example, in key journals – could 'make me feel anxious,' said one doctor, with the result that: 'With me messing about with his medication and trying to practise evidence-based medicine, I found it was making him [the patient] feel more anxious.'

When discussing the process of coming to a decision, the doctors in this study clearly held the view that their choice of words in consultations could sway patients to accept or reject clinical evidence. Doctors realise this, and can use it to pre-empt patients' decisions. 'It's how you put it over,' said one group member. 'It depends on how you feed information to people,' said another. Finally, although the evidence might be strong, and its relevance in certain cases clear, logistics could still act as a barrier. Referring to the anxiety about a patient bleeding while on warfarin (a recognised side-effect of this drug), one practitioner remarked that: 'It's not a minor bleed if your patient is 30 miles from the nearest transfusion service.'

Conclusion

These general practitioner participants appeared to act as a conduit within the consultation and to regard clinical evidence as a square peg to be fitted in the round hole of the patient's life. The process of implementation is complex, fluid and adaptive.

Commentary on why general practitioners do not implement the evidence: a qualitative study

This study was prompted by two conversations. The first arose from a discussion about the study by McColl *et al.* (1998) referred to in the introductory section of the paper. This paper had suggested that there may be unique reasons within a general practice setting that might constitute barriers to the implementation of evidence-based medicine. The second conversation, which followed from this, was a further exploration of the notion of personal significance referred to earlier. If there were unique barriers to implementing evidence-based medicine, what might they be? Could they be partly explained by the idea underpinning personal significance, namely the opaque activity of transferring ideas from professional to patient, and vice versa? The area remained under-researched, and this study held out the possibility of extending the findings of the preliminary study published in the previous year and presented as Paper 2 in this chapter (Mears and Sweeney, 2000).

Commentary on the data

The data that appeared in the final published draft of this paper provided a fair and accurate reflection of the analysis of the original focus groups' transcripts. The editors of the *BMJ* requested a redrafting of the discussion section of the paper, but were happy with the presentation of the results as we had initially suggested. No further elaboration of the results is required here.

Summary

The main findings of this study extend and support the relevance of personal significance to clinical practice. One observes the practitioners distilling clinical evidence internally, as it were, weighing it up against their own experience, both personal and professional. One senses that, having come to a view themselves, the doctors know that they can – and indeed have to – 'sell' that view to their patients, in the context of an elaborate, fluid, and evolving relationship to which both parties – the patient and the doctor – contribute. And all of this proceeds against a background of anxiety created by the very presence of the evidence (in 'all the *BMJ*s, all the rags'), as well as the logistical challenges inherent in its implementation. These observations will be developed during the second-level analysis at the end of this chapter.

Paper 4

A comparison of professionals' and patients' understanding of asthma: evidence of emerging dualities?

Published in 2001 in *Journal of Medical Ethics: Medical Humanities.* **27**: 20–25.[6]

Background

The purpose of this paper was to extend the debate about the nature of medicine's explanatory model, which had been developed in the first three papers, into the patient's domain. The first paper tentatively explored whether, when discussing the nature of clinical practice in the context of joint working, health and social care professionals expressed some views about the deeper nature of clinical practice and the context in which they practised. The next two papers collated empirical data about 'personal significance', the nature of which is described in Chapter 5. This final paper focuses on another aspect of personal significance, which is enshrined in the reciprocity that lies at the heart of its definition. At stake is the debate about modelling a disease – in this case asthma – on the basis of a biomedical model predicated on scientific positivism. If the contemporary explanatory model was to dominate clinical discussions, one might expect a reasonable degree of sharedness of that understanding, the absence of which could constitute an impediment to joint 'shared' decision making. This is what this paper explores.

Method

Two sets of focus groups were convened in parallel, four consisting of professionals (doctors and nurses) and four comprising patients with asthma. The professional groups consisted of one separate group each of specialist doctors, secondary care nurses, general practitioners and practice nurses. Patients with asthma were identified from general practice disease registers. To obtain a sufficient spread of patients with the type of asthma that is seen routinely in general practice, the sampling frame was stratified by age and by use of inhaled steroids (which was used as a proxy indicator of asthma severity).

Main results

The healthcare professionals and patients who participated in this study showed broad agreement in their explanations of the aetiology and drug treatment of asthma. However, the data suggest a lack of congruence in the development of treatment strategies and locus of control. In summary, the doctors and nurses constructed management plans *prospectively* – based, for example, on their theoretical knowledge of the effects of inhaled steroids over time. When referring to Ventolin and Becotide (standard symptomatic and prophylactic treatments, respectively, for asthma), one general practitioner said: 'one makes you better at the time, the other keeps you better for tomorrow.' The patients formulated such plans *retrospectively*, based on their previous experience of various treatment modalities. For example, a younger male patient who frequently used an inhaler

---

[6] Authors: KG Sweeney, K Edwards, J Stead and D Halpin, University of Exeter and North and East Devon Health Authority.

said: 'I take it if I get bad or get a cold . . . on to my browns three or four days then it works. All the bad stuff comes towards it and bounces off it or gets eaten possibly. Maybe absorbed.' This sometimes led individuals to act against medical advice to use Becotide continuously: 'When you haven't got a tight chest you haven't got asthma. I just forget to take Becotide' (older male patient who was an infrequent inhaler user).

The healthcare professionals and patients in this study used different metaphors to conceptualise asthma. The former group more frequently used metaphors that evoked ongoing processes. Consider, for example, this doctor's comment: 'it involves probably formal components of your inflammatory pathway, so probably certain parts can be switched off . . . some are more prominent than others.' Compare that with the following lay participants' models, which represent the tendency of the patients to visualise the chest (in their use of metaphor) as a static container, emptying and filling throughout the course of the disease: 'It's like a windsock' (younger, infrequent user) and 'hubbly-bubbly pipes' (younger, frequent user).

Conclusion

The analysis supports the view that there is an epistemological difference between doctors and patients in this context. We postulate that the two groups – professionals and patients – draw on different types of knowledge when constructing their model of asthma. Doctors, it is asserted, draw more on theoretical knowledge, whereas patients make use of their lived experience, drawing on what Piaget (1932) calls 'figurative knowledge.'

Comment on the data

Very few constraints were placed on the presentation of the data by the editors of this journal. The published paper was 4500 words in length.

Summary

There does not appear to be a single, uniform conceptualisation of asthma that was shared and explored by the professionals and patients in this study. If the biomedical model, in this case of asthma, predicated on scientific positivism, was indeed hegemonic, and constituted the dominant currency in discussions, one might reasonably expect, if not an equivalence, at least a conspicuous degree of overlap. We observe here an ongoing tension between two different types of knowledge – referred to as operational (theory based) and figurative (derived from lived experience) – which, the paper argues, suggests that the two groups are drawing on different epistemological frameworks. This theme will be elaborated when the second-level analysis reflects on the relevance of complex responsive processes to clinical conversations.

Second-level analysis of the papers

In this section, the main themes distilled from the four papers presented in this chapter are analysed from the perspective of complex adaptive systems. The five key features of complex adaptive systems, which were set out earlier in this chapter, are held as the compass points for the analytical framework.

Preliminary observations on the data collection in the four papers

As the four papers presented in this chapter represent 'one-off' data collection exercises – snapshots, as it were, of the experiences reported – they are unlikely to yield primary evidence of features of complex systems that evolve over time. Time-series data, which collect evidence at various points throughout the evolution of a system, would be more likely to achieve that (Holt, 2002b). Thus one would not expect to see primary evidence of self-organisation and co-evolution which, de facto, occur over time. Participants may refer to these features of complex systems when they describe the context in which they were operating, thus providing some indirect evidence of their influence. The other two features of complex systems, namely receptive context (also termed enabling context; Mitelton-Kelly, 2003) and complex responsive processes, are more likely to be identified.

Given the criteria for a complex system that were set out in Chapter 5, one can then postulate that there should be evidence of the presence of an enabling framework in systems which evolved creatively, or evidence of its absence in more dysfunctional systems. And if complex responsive processes are fundamental to human adaptive systems, one should discern evidence of these, or at least reference to them. Thus this second-level analysis is undertaken tentatively in relation to these four papers, as the research that they report was not conducted primarily with the two-level analysis in mind (Sweeney, 2003b).

Receptive context

Consider the definition of receptive context that was presented in Chapter 5. It embraced the following notions:

- an enabling framework, or an infrastructure of communicability
- a set of conditions that have the potential to facilitate the development of complex conversations and actions, whose patterning can, over time, constitute a complex system
- a set of values through which coherent action can be expressed
- the presence of leadership to initiate complex responsive processes
- the potential to engage other agents to co-create and adapt the system.

In Paper 1 (on joint working), we are told in the background information that the study day on evidence-based medicine was held on behalf of a community in which there was little evidence of joint working in the context of evidence-based medicine. We learn that the participants bemoan their inability to secure meetings at which all the 'right people' turn up, and that their quite distinct – indeed opposing – views on what constitutes the medical and social models reduced their enthusiasm for joint working. So did the physical location, which they described as 'out here', evoking a feeling of being marginalised, and peripheral to a more central place where financial decisions were made. Some of the participants saw evidence-based practice, which was considered as one mechanism for facilitating joint working, as a threat, making them realise that they had been 'doing something futile for 20 years.'

This constitutes evidence which suggests the absence of a receptive context, or that the participants were not operating within an enabling framework. I postulate the existence of a link between the absence of such a framework and the absence of coherent action, leadership to encourage it, and other agents enthusiastically co-creating it. This hypothesis is supported by the evidence describing the barriers to joint working, and makes sense in the light of the reason for holding the study day in the first place. Given the criteria for a complex system that were described in Chapter 5, one concludes that the system in which the participants in this study operated – a health and social care 'community' – was not complex or adaptive.

A similar analysis can be applied to the background to Paper 4 (on asthma). The background to this paper involves the recognition that, despite a clearer under-standing of the pathogenesis of asthma and an increase in services provided to patients with the condition, morbidity and mortality remain high. We learn in the paper that, although both professionals and patients agree about the basics of what causes the disease, there is less congruence of opinion about how to manage it, particularly with regard to the role of inhaled steroids. Locus of control is also disputed, with a tacit assumption among many of the healthcare professionals that they can delegate control to patients (implying its prior location within their sphere of influence). The patients' response is typified by the comment made by one sufferer that: 'I know my asthma better than anybody.' The analysis at the end of the paper supports the deployment of different epistemological frame-works by the two participating groups.

There is no direct evidence in this paper that links morbidity in these patients to the absence of a shared understanding of asthma or its management, but one can speculate about such an association. Accepting the features of receptive context described above, one is led to conclude that there is evidence of some but not all the features of an enabling framework. The set of conditions, namely the professional–patient interactions described in the paper, have at least the potential to construct an enabling framework, and one can infer from the participants' reports that the two groups shared some values – for example, the desire to manage asthma successfully. However, against this the presence of two different models for the disease, reflecting the deployment of operational and figurative knowledge, does not support the presence of a shared, complementary set of values through which complex conversations may lead to coherent action. And there is no evidence in the study that the interactions between the professionals and the patients satisfied the description of complex responsive responses. The nature of any leadership associated with the initiation of coherent action is disputed. Who is to lead – the patient or the doctor? Thus one can conclude that although there is some evidence of some of the features of a receptive context, one cannot confidently discern its presence and its influence on the evolution of the system, which consequently cannot be described as complex or adaptive on the basis of this evidence.

Second-level analysis of Papers 2 and 3

In this section, the second-level analysis of Papers 2 and 3 focuses on the three features that together constitute the minimum conditions necessary for a system to be considered complex and adaptive.

Complex responsive processes in Papers 2 and 3

The definition of a complex responsive process that is offered by Stacey (2001) suggests that:

- it involves interaction through complex communication
- one participant issues a gesture, which in turn calls forth a response from the other, in an iterative, interactive process
- this interaction is self-organising, and has the property of emergent coherence
- the nature of such processes has the potential to be transformational. In participating in a complex responsive process, the conversation is changed, each participant is changed, the nature of their relationship can change, and by a ripple effect, the nature of the participants' relationship with the larger system can change
- these processes are inherently unpredictable.

There is some evidence to support the presence of complex responsive processes in both Papers 2 and 3, which for the purposes of this second-level analysis are considered together, as they explore similar systems, namely the doctor–patient dyad. The notion of a gesture calling forth a response is supported by the description of conversations by one of the participants in Paper 2, who commented that: 'You can make a remark, or a question which shows you're on line, then you're away . . . similarly if you ask a question which shows you're not, they'll stay dumb and blocked.' Indeed, patients 'shop around' to select doctors with whom they can conduct these delicate exchanges of gesture and response. The doctors in this study agreed that 'you have to know where patients are coming from, what their beliefs are . . .'. In the context of complex responsive processes, this is a prerequisite of an enabling framework within which such creative conversations can take place. These relationships, expressed through complex conversations, 'continue and go on', and need preserving in order to mature – hence the flexibility to concede on trivial issues, such as the occasional penicillin prescription.

Did the participants in these two studies declare that they might be changed themselves in the process of these conversations? It seems so. 'We are influenced at least as much, if not more,' asserted one general practitioner in Paper 3, 'by the experience of individual patients as we are by the evidence.' Did the nature of their conversation change in the course of their evolution? The evidence does not dispute this. One doctor, we learn, built up the relationship with the patient by initially not following the guidelines, and then, when they were in a position of greater trust, they were able to implement the guidelines. 'I have followed the guidelines, of course,' this doctor stated, 'but in a sneaky way, and it's taken about three months to do it.' Accordingly, one can cautiously conclude that the interactions which these participants were describing were complex responsive processes.

Receptive context and self-organisation in Papers 2 and 3

Is there evidence from the first-level analysis of these two papers to support the presence of a receptive context? In Table 7.1 the five features of receptive context are shown in the left-hand column, with a second-level commentary for each feature in the right-hand column.

In order to qualify as a complex and adaptive system, we have agreed that three features should be evidenced, namely a receptive context, complex responsive processes and self-organisation. When analysing these papers, which reflect 'one-off' snapshots of a system, it will be difficult to discern evidence of the last of this triad, namely self-organisation. However, some preliminary observations can be made.

Self-organisation is about the creation of coherent patterns of behaviour. One can speculate from the doctors' descriptions in these two papers that there are some patterns to the behaviours that were acted out in their consultations with patients.

Table 7.1 Receptive context in Papers 2 and 3

Feature of receptive context	Comment on evidence in Papers 2 and 3
Infrastructure of communicability	The nature of the consultations to which they refer suggests the presence of an appropriate infrastructure in which the doctor–patient dyad has the potential to evolve
A set of conditions to promote complex responsive processes	There is some indirect evidence from the doctors of the influence of their previous experiences on evolving relationships. They also refer to patients' beliefs as an important component of their interaction
A set of values for coherent action to be expressed	The data imply an aspiration that the doctors provide, and the patients receive, the best possible care. In their interaction with patients, the doctors refer to their own philosophy of health, and the way patients develop their own beliefs about health and disease. Although there is no direct evidence linking these to coherent action, the conditions for such action may be said to be present
The presence of leadership to initiate complex responsive processes	There is indirect evidence of this. The doctors appeared to be disinclined to apply the rules of evidence-based medicine slavishly, and they acknowledged that sometimes patients lead (e.g. in cases where the patient doesn't believe that a treatment will work). This evokes the notion of dispersed leadership described by Durie *et al.* (2004)
The potential to engage other agents to co-create and adapt the system	One can infer that other agents influence the nature of the interactions between doctors and participants. The doctors refer to 'society', and one can assume that the patients' beliefs are created within their own life worlds in which they interact with significant others

Thus they talk of 'knowing where the patients are coming from', and of the evidence being 'tempered by the patient and the doctor.' One participant describes implementing guidelines in a 'sneaky' way, which implies some form of pattern in a series of interactions that are spread over time. More broadly, the doctors refer to a continuously changing, moulding and evolving relationship with their patients, whose patterning allows some decisions to be taken which, although not technically justifiable (like the prescription of an antibiotic), are deployed in order to maintain the pattern of communication (the ongoing relationship with that patient).

Thus one can conclude that there is some evidence to support the view that the participants in these two studies did operate within a receptive context, and that the nature of their interaction satisfied the definition of complex responsive processes. The evidence for self-organisation is much less clear, is indirect, and is based on inferences that were made on the basis of the participants' descriptions.

Summary of second-level analysis

It must be emphasised that this second-level analysis is undertaken with great caution as, at the point of data collection, no attention was paid to the possibility of collating material that could directly support (or dispute) the relevance of these features of complex adaptive systems.

In Paper 1 (on joint working) there are enough data for it to be accepted that a receptive context was not present, and that consequently the system under scrutiny was not complex. One can speculate that the absence of a receptive context might have been related to the reason for holding the study day to which the participants contributed, namely the absence of good collaborative working between local health and social care professionals. In Paper 4 (the asthma study) only some of the features of a receptive context are supported, and it is not clear that the nature of the interaction between the professional and patient groups constituted a set of complex responsive processes. One could have collected data that might have clarified the nature of these interactions, but the data as presented do not allow this.

However, there is stronger although inconclusive evidence for the presence of complex adaptive systems operating in the interactions described in Papers 2 and 3. The interactions appear to constitute complex responsive processes, and there is some, albeit indirect evidence of a receptive context. Although there is not clear prima facie evidence of self-organisation, one can cautiously make some inferences about this from the descriptions given by the participating doctors. This analysis permits further reflection on the notion of personal significance (described in Chapter 3).

Given what is now understood about the nature and importance of complex responsive processes, personal significance may actually consist, at its root, of such complex processes. Personal significance can be considered as the emergent property of the patterning of complex responsive processes. Overall, the analysis supports the view that further research looking more directly for evidence of complex systems might usefully be undertaken.

Summary: reflections on second-level analysis and the direction of future research

The main purpose of exploring these four small studies was to illustrate how the principles of complexity might be incorporated into a usable research methodology, and to demonstrate what kind of conclusions one might draw using this method, and given the definitions of the features of complex and evolving systems set out in Chapter 5. In short, it appears to be possible to deploy the principles of complexity as an interpretive framework at a second level, once a conventional first-level analysis of collated data has been undertaken using the basic principles of qualitative research. Although there is always a danger of reading into the data to gather evidence from this interpretive framework, this is a danger inherent in any focused qualitative analysis. Marxist, feminist or racial perspectives are perfectly acceptable frameworks to deploy in qualitative analysis, and they run the same risk. In this example, one takes the principles of complex systems and scrutinises the assembled themes for data which constitute evidence that they were or were not in place. One cannot create evidence to support such conclusions, but one can identify such evidence and comment on its merits.

So what kind of domains might benefit from the kind of second-level analysis set out above? Inherent in the notion of complex adaptive systems is time – time for the systems to evolve and mature, expressing, over time, characteristic features through the patterning of iterative processes that give rise to the system's emergent properties through self-organisation and co-evolution. This gives us a clue as to which topics might benefit from such an analysis.

Accordingly, the principles of complexity may usefully be deployed in researching programmes of organisational change in healthcare systems. Complexity could be used to understand the challenges to clinical practice, which involve a cultural or work practice change – for example, the implementation of a National Service Framework, or the introduction of a new technology. And a framework based on the principles of complex adaptive systems could form the basis of an assessment of major shifts in the deployment of human resources in healthcare – for example, the impact of the work of general practitioners with a special interest, or the impact of employing nurses as first-contact care clinicians in primary care.

In addition, complexity may be a useful framework for gaining a clearer understanding of patients' narratives (Snowden, 2002). Here the use of a reflective diary which is updated iteratively over time, and which recounts in detail the chronological sequence of events in an illness experience, could be analysed from a complexity perspective in order to understand how the patient interacted with the system, and how the system responded, affording opportunities to reflect on the evolution of the system over time. In future studies in which the perspective of complexity is to be applied, it will be useful to collect participants' stories, as they may shed light on the nature of the evolving processes that constitute the system under scrutiny, and they may also illustrate how interactions within those systems come to be patterned in a particular way.

In the previous chapter I discussed the opportunities afforded to healthcare by the developments in non-linear mathematics for understanding change in some physiological and pathological systems. Although the details of the mathematics involved are beyond the scope of the non-specialist, it is appropriate to speculate how our understanding of the evolution of pathological systems over time can be assisted by these developments. It is likely, as Holt (2002a) argues, that models of diabetes based on non-linear mathematics will help patients to manage that condition better; and Tennison (2002) argues that we will be able to understand the cyclical infectivity of some pathogens by drawing on non-linear mathematics.

In summary, the principles of complexity can assist healthcare research in domains of transformational change, whether that change occurs in organisations, in cultural shifts in clinical practice, or in the narrative recounting of illness experiences. So far as human physiological and pathological systems are concerned, the ability to collate accurate numerical data over time opens the interpretation of these systems to the benefits of non-linear mathematics. I shall develop these themes in the next and final chapter.

Chapter 8

Complexity and medical practice: prospects for the future

Introduction

There really is only one question to address when evaluating the potential benefits of utilising the principles of complexity in healthcare: will this make me a better doctor? Related to this is the form of the question at the organisational level: will understanding complexity make ours a better health service? In turn, this invites the same question at a clinical level: will this make us better clinicians? This chapter will attempt to answer these questions.

Asking questions

What the preceding chapters have done is to ask questions *about* the questions that doctors ask. First, we have asked how we know things in medicine. We have an explanatory model, I have argued, that is rooted in scientific positivism. This link between the explanatory model and its related world-view (or ontological perspective) has been explored, to argue that a world-view is expressed in a predilection for a certain type of knowledge, which we have called an epistemological perspective. When we speculate that this triumvirate, ontological perspective, epistemological framework and explanatory model might serve as a generic model, we are permitted to ask whether there are other ways of knowing, expressed in different types of knowledge, leading to distinct explanatory models. I have argued that the naturalistic tradition is predicated on a world-view that differs from scientific positivism and that deploys a socially constructed epistemology, from which has arisen an explanatory model that concerns itself with attitudes and beliefs, with intention and action. One way in which this is used in healthcare is through the principles of qualitative research.

In Chapter 3 we reflected on the contemporary form of the explanatory model in medicine, by setting out the principles of evidence-based medicine, and then reminding ourselves of the criticisms that it had attracted. At the outset, one could be forgiven for asking why a model which simply exhorted practitioners to apply the best evidence to solve clinical questions, and in so doing equipped those same practitioners with useful critical skills, could attract such an enthusiastic critique. The answer lay in the nature of the critics' concerns. First, evidence-based medicine involves an initial abstraction – an extraction of a suitable biomedical question from the patient's narrative. If a story of sleeplessness, fear, uncertainty and malaise is called 'anxiety', then the hounds are out on the course, and the search for best evidence can proceed – we have a 'case' for valium. If a naturalistic interpretation is applied, an array of personal, behavioural and structural impediments to well-being is exposed, leading to a different strategy for resolution. These interpretations are not mutually exclusive, and good clinicians will pursue both. However, in so doing we have supported the key proposition in the first part of this book, namely that there is more than one way of knowing. Good clinicians will deploy two ontological views, and in turn will seek out the preferred knowledge to populate each view.

Mrs B's consultation showed us how this can happen in the most mundane of consultations. Here we had an intersection of ways of knowing, a clash of the positivist and naturalistic ways of knowing. What happens, we can ask, when such a clash occurs? Does one view dominate? If so, who decides which view does dominate? And if some coalition of world-views is to be fashioned, by whom is that coalition created? This raises two questions about the nature of these common but profound consultations. First, where does the locus of control lie in these consultations? Is it always driven by the doctor, an assumption driven by a conventional understanding of the doctor as expert? Or is it more desirable to see the role of the doctor as that of the informed servant, like the butler in the *Death of Ivan Illyich*, supporting, informing and guiding the patient towards their own decision which suits the particularities of the context rather than the generalities of the evidence? The second question is when is enough, enough? The fact that many individuals in middle or late-middle age are surviving what a mere decade and a half ago would have been a fatal clinical event means that they survive into later life, susceptible to a constellation of comorbid conditions which develop as a consequence of their longevity. Mrs B is an example of this. Her comorbidity was amenable to treatment of all of its constituent conditions (with the possible exception of her macular degeneration). In that consultation, I offered evidence to support tighter control of her blood pressure, her glycosylated haemoglobin and her dyslipidaemia, and could have justified more active intervention for her intercurrent depression and background arthropathy. In her historic riposte, 'Jack's dead and the boys have gone', she asked the question which will challenge the next generation of practitioners more than my own generation: when is enough, enough? We are encountering a new kind of coercive public health, where 'health' is seen as a minority sport. Around 90% of the adult European population, we learn, is now considered to be 'at risk' of cardiovascular disease. Virtually the entire continental population will be asked to submit to monitoring, to vigilant personal surveillance and often to medical intervention. It is when we articulate our response to that challenge that we must begin to ask questions about the questions that doctors ask.

None of this is really new. Thus presented, in the context of complexity, the observations are a restatement, and a contemporary attempt to address the age-old problem, for clinicians, of balancing the general with the particular. With the advent of evidence-based medicine, clinicians were encouraged to interpolate from population data to individuals. In so doing, however, we were at the mercy of the ecological fallacy – assuming that any and all conclusions derived from population data could be applied to all individuals in the data set. A number of attempts have been made over the years to integrate these two seemingly irreconcilable perspectives. Greenhalgh (2002) has called for intuition in general practice. She describes this as the rapid, unconscious process of integrating multiple complex pieces of data, where causality is set aside and selective attention is paid to fine detail. Importantly, clinicians become increasingly skilled at exercising intuition over time, re-establishing the importance of experience, or what Aristotle would call phronesis (wisdom) in the process (Ross, 1988). More recently, Gillies (2005) has described deliberative specification as the means of synthesising evidence and intuition. This allows Gillies to accord appropriate but proportional weight to the evidence, while also paying attention to the unique particularities of the patient's context. The contribution of the principles of complexity is to extend our ability to theorise about how, in practice, this process of deliberative speculation might express itself. In the notion of complex responsive processes, we have a model of communication that confirms the continuous, subtle co-evolution of the relationship between doctor and patient. Note the use of the term 'co-evolution', which implies that both participants are changed during the process of their interaction. Doctors are not immune from this change as a result of their status, but are both contributors to and alumni of that change process. It is in that iterative and recursive interaction, leading to change, that we find the roots of the experience at the heart of intuition. Complexity helps us not just by legitimising, theoretically, the need to reconcile evidence and context, but also by showing how pervasive and inevitable that process is. No matter how good the evidence, or how sound the clinician's judgement, if the patient is not engaged in a meaningful, changing interaction, they will count for nothing. Ultimately, in the clinical encounter, it is the patient who decides what the nature of the outcome will be, through either concordance or its absence. A new metaphor is needed to describe this relationship between doctor and patient – the doctor as the informed servant.

The principles of complexity, set alongside the analyses in the preceding chapters, tell us one thing above all, namely that there are several ways of knowing. Doctors, I argue, deploy not one but a whole range of ontological perspectives when they consult, drawing on a range of epistemological frameworks to populate their explanations. In general practice, above all, it is important not to let one perspective form the unique basis of the interaction. Attention to particularities, recognition of uniqueness, and a greater willingness to accept intuition as an asset that matures with age, combine to encourage flexibility in the consultation and a recognition that we, as clinicians, are ourselves part of that change process, and will be subtly affected by it. This is the framework within which the three dimensions of generalism were presented in the introduction to this book. Technical generalism is the conventional understanding of the skills of the general practitioner – the ability to deploy diagnostic and managerial skills over a wide range of the partialist specialisms of secondary care. Contextual generalism conveys the importance of a second dimension, recognising that the dynamic of a consultation can change profoundly and swiftly. Drawing on the principles of complexity, we can theorise that it is in recursive interaction of complex responsive processes within the consultation that such contextual changes occur, and are recognised and legitimised. Now we can understand that evidentiary generalism is a third dimension which is implied by the first two, namely the need to understand that when context shifts in a consultation, the index paradigm and its related epistemological framework shift, too. The generalist, drawing on the skills of evidentiary generalism, recognises the legitimacy of utilising a range of evidentiary frameworks, will come to an understanding with the patient about the balance of the biomedical with the biographical, and will be prepared to accept, in certain circumstances, the supremacy of the latter over the former. It is when that balance is appropriately struck that both participants in the consultation will feel able to answer this key question for twenty-first century medicine: when is enough, enough?

Complexity and science

Heisenberg more than anyone tells us how dramatically science changed in the second half of the twentieth century. 'The ground,' he wrote, 'was being cut from underneath science' (Heisenberg, 1971). Linearity gave way to non-linearity; reductionism gave way to relationality, and unidirectional algorithm gave way to recursive dynamic. In mathematics, the discovery of non-integer dimensions, the Lyapunov exponent and period doubling provided a deeper understanding of poorly understood areas, broadening the applicability of non-linear mathematics to thermodynamics, biology, ecology and geology. Of great interest was the discovery of the seemingly universal Feigenbaum's number, which describes the period-doubling interval in recursive systems in a huge and disparate array of disciplines. Feigenbaum's constant began to look like the 'pi' (22/7, or π, written in Greek) of non-linearity. And autocatalysis, the process whereby the presence of one particular chemical encourages its own production via positive feedback, had far-reaching effects in the field of developmental biology. Within the last two decades, actuator chemicals (which encourage autocatalysis) and inhibitor chemicals (which discourage that process) have been shown to be involved in the evolution of the markings on the skin and coat of mammals (Gribbin, 2004). The implications of non-linear systems for developmental biology are still being debated.

Many commentators (Capra, 1983; Stewart, 1989) have argued that these new insights provided the impetus for the affected disciplines to revisit their explanatory models. However, it was not as if the *ancien régime* of linearity had been expelled and replaced. Rather, a new relationship between linear and non-linear systems was evolving, based on the mathematical relationship between the two, namely that the former was a special case of the latter. Had chaos and complexity simply provided a new set of metaphors for these disciplines, or had something more profound, radical and permanent happened to their explanatory models? Although it is beyond the scope of this book to make that judgement, the pervasiveness of Feigenbaum's constant, and the curious way in which simple non-linear modelling seems to be applicable over a wide range of very disparate disciplines, hints at something more than a useful set of metaphors. The work on catalysis referred to above (by Turing in computing) was quickly applied to inorganic chemistry (by Lotka), then to predator–prey populations (by Volterra), and then to thermodynamics (by Belousov, Zhabotinsky and finally Prigogine) (Gribbin, 2004). Although none of this spread occurred logically or predictably (Turing, Lotka and Volterra were all dead when Belousov first reported, and had dismissed, his findings in 1951), the consequence in terms of revising the explanatory model was profound – an acknowledgement that some modification to the second law of thermodynamics was needed when systems operating far from equilibrium were being explored.

In clinical medicine, we are already witnessing the benefits of exploring physiological systems through the mathematics of chaos. New understanding is emerging about the physiology of the heart, with speculation that pathological processes might be the result of the loss of the chaotic features that seem to characterise normal function. It looks as if respiratory and renal physiology demonstrate similar fractal properties, and new applications of the principles of chaos theory are likely to produce fresh insights into these systems. In addition, for nearly a decade now epidemiologists have been applying these principles in order to obtain a clearer understanding of the incidence of a range of diseases (Tennison, 2002).

Although it is difficult to see how these principles might be applied to the commoner chronic diseases in general practice, one can make a number of observations. First, it is likely that research into diabetes will reveal its chaotic properties (Holt T, 2005, personal communication). This kind of research will require new types of data collection. Real-time data sets, providing thousands of data inputs over a long period of time, will be needed to enable researchers to see the patterning in such systems. 'N of 1' trials may become more relevant to clinical practice in primary care, as a practical step towards synthesising observations made during population studies with the unique make-up of the individual patient. To this end, Bayesian statistical methods might serve us better than probabilistic models.

Complexity and organisations

Although the mathematics of chaos opened up new vistas for the quantitative sciences, in the last quarter of the twentieth century the principles of complexity were increasingly being applied in order to understand how large organisations operated and changed. Several examples that show how the principles of complex and adapting systems have helped us to understand how a change process has worked have been given in Chapter 6. From this and other research currently being undertaken within the National Health Service in the UK, we can begin to make a number of observations about the value of these principles for such research.

Ultimately, what seems crucial to the implementation and maintenance of change is the iterative interaction that is the basis of complex responsive processes – those processes whereby the participants in an interaction change subtly over time, their conversation changes, then their interaction with other agents in the system subtly changes and, by a ripple effect, the system itself changes. Now this might seem obvious (and it is), but complexity allows us to theorise as to why this might be. In the course of these iterative interactions, the key element that changes is the relationship between the participants. The examples given in Chapter 6, together with current NHS research, suggest that it is by the forming of new relationships (and, by implication, the discarding of old ones) that an agenda can move forward. First, these new relationships must be predicated on an agreement that 'things in the system' have to change. Leaders, for example, have to lead in a different way, dispersing their authority in a manner that, unnervingly perhaps, gives them less control, but which liberates significant others to operate more authoritatively within the system. Secondly, the creating of these new relationships has to be a conscious decision, not an unplanned elaboration of a pre-existing relationship. Thirdly, part of the conscious decision involves self-realisation, an acceptance, or better a discovery that an agenda has to, and can, move forward – the 'penny-dropping' moment, if you like. This analysis helps us understand why change imposed from outside a system is often unsuccessful. Unless those participating in a system first accept that things have to change, and secondly discover for themselves how change might occur, the change process will not constitute a visceral part of their interaction. Think of how 'gaming' happens in organisations – the response to change which accommodates it, according to some rules of engagement, but with no internal acceptance of its need or value.

A second insight that is provided by the principles of complex systems involves the notion of 'adjacent possibles' (Durie R, 2004, personal communication). Adjacent possibles are notional 'spaces' in which change can occur, as a consequence of interaction between the agents in a system, leading to self-organisation. These spaces can be said to be 'adjacent' in that they are within organisational reach for the participants, that is not too different to destabilise the system, but sufficiently different to encourage change, initially usually on a small scale. Such changes, if successful, can then be patterned over the system to create change on a wider scale. The opposite of this is also true – if they are unsuccessful, but on a small scale, they do not destabilise the system, although they don't change it either. Consider, as a theoretical example, a healthcare community that wants to set up a primary-care-based, intermediate service for a chronic disease, such as diabetes. The idea of adjacent possibles suggests that such a change should be sufficiently within the organisation 'reach' of all the significant participants in the system, but sufficiently different to constitute a change (in the form of an improvement) in the provision when established. In planning such a change process, one must first accept the possibility of failure, as unless the system is coerced into changing, the agents will, through their own interaction, determine the outcome of the process themselves. Secondly, one sees the need to engage all potentially significant participants early on, if only to initiate the interaction, and hopefully to assist in the co-creation of some complex responsive processes, through the sharing of common values and aspirations, which constitute the receptive context of the system at its outset. Any programme of change should then be small enough to be discernibly different, while not destabilising the system if it fails. In the example of an enhanced diabetes service, this might look like joint working between primary and secondary care providers in a locality, or through a cluster of general practices, which, if successful, could be patterned subsequently through the wider health and social care community. The change would then be 'adjacent' organisationally, and 'possible' inter-professionally. What would *not* constitute an adjacent possible would be the unilateral establishment of a stand-alone intermediate service, no matter how well provided, as it would have failed to engage the key players, and it would run the risk of failing to be patterned – that is, accepted by the local community. One can theorise that, in the setting up of these adjacent possibles, the planning might have to be quite linear. In the diabetes example, this might involve the decision to set up the service to serve, say, a specific number of patients over a specific, short period of time, with an agreed set of actions to be provided and reviewed – for example, to manage 30 patients from three practices for one year (an agreed interval for a full diabetic review) and scrutinise the clinical and patient-based outcomes. At that point, if successful, the patterning of the change, in the form of its wider adoption by the whole community, might flow in a less controlled, non-linear way, allowing the participants to self-organise around a small number of agreed strategic values. It might also co-evolve, as needed, with systems either nested within that community (other general practices) or outside the immediate system (national bodies or other healthcare communities).

Summary

The main proposition in this book is about ways of knowing. I have argued that, by exploring the glorious intellectual history of western civilisation, one discerns a trend which gave rise to the scientific positivism at the heart of the clinical method, and a parallel trend, described as naturalistic, from which a more grounded understanding of the human condition arose, and out of which the principles of what we now call qualitative research emerged. In the last third of the twentieth century, many of the fundamental sciences – thermodynamics and biology in particular – revised their explanatory models to accommodate the insights provided through the principles of chaos and complexity. These insights, which were presented in Chapters 5 and 6, have implications for medicine. At the clinical level, the applications of the mathematical models of chaos are yielding new understanding of physiology. At the organisational level, the principles of complex and adapting systems are helping us to understand how large organisations work. This in turn will help us to understand how policy might be better crafted, how change might be better shaped, and how uncertainty is an inescapable (and perhaps healthy) part of that process. At the theoretical level, chaos and complexity can help us to synthesise evidence and intuition. They dignify the notion of intuition, and re-establish the importance of experience and wisdom, seeing them as emergent properties of the thousands of iterative, recursive interactions in consultations. Are chaos and complexity the answer to life, the universe and everything? Probably not, but they do help us to ask better questions about the questions that doctors ask.

Appendix

Paper 1

Kieran Sweeney

LECTURER IN GENERAL PRACTICE
AND HEALTH SERVICES RESEARCH,
EXETER UNIVERSITY

Jonathan Stead
Liz Cosford

NORTH AND EAST DEVON
HEALTH AUTHORITY

research into practice

Evidence-Based Practice: Can This Help Joint Working?

ABSTRACT

This article presents a qualitative analysis of three focus groups convened during a study day for health and social care professionals, which reveals a strong perception of a philosophical difference in approaches to professional practice.

The prospect of health and social care professionals working more closely together is welcomed, and evidence-based practice should be encouraged and financially supported.

While established educational strategies can be deployed to respond to the conventional perceived barriers to working together, more innovative models are needed. The authors commend the model of Significant Event Auditing.

Introduction: collaboration and evidence-based care

Collaboration is the new deity in health and social care. Encouraging the two groups of professions to work together is politically correct, professionally desirable and likely to lead to greater integration in the delivery of health and social care services. Actually, the mantra of collaboration has been sounded for over three decades, but advocating working together has been a lot easier than realising it in the field (Clarke, 2000). A myriad of impediments have been cited to explain this failure, the three most frequent reasons being differing professional perspectives on problems, different occupational cultures and confusion over professional roles (Sheldon, 1994; Dalley, 1991; Abramson & Mizrahi, 1996). Leedham and Wistow (1992) argued that differences in values between general practitioners and social workers actually produced conflict which undermined the best-laid plans for collaboration.

Both health and social services are also required to deliver evidence-based care. Could training in evidence-based practice through acquiring critical appraisal skills achieve what other strategies have so far failed to do? There is little direct evidence to raise hopes, but many policy-makers have identified joint training as a means through which many of the impediments to joint working could be overcome (Department of Health/Social Services Inspectorate, 1991). Training together would dispel mistrust, Gambetta (1998) argued, and governments tend to agree (Department of Health/Social Services Inspectorate, 1989).

research into practice

This article reports on a joint study day held in April 1998 which provided an opportunity for health and social care professionals in one locality to express their views on joint working, in the context of a joint training exercise in evidence-based practice. A group of professionals from health and social care were invited to attend a study day to discuss the principles of evidence-based practice, to receive an introduction to critical appraisal skills and to reflect on perceived barriers to working together. As part of the study day, three small groups of mixed professionals were convened for one hour, during which their views on these topics were explored and recorded. Efforts were made to continue with the groups in their localities after the study day. This report presents the analysis of the data collated from these groups, postulates some theory to explain the analysis and offers a strategy for acting on the findings.

Methodology

Following a formal presentation on critical appraisal skills, three focus groups (Morgan, 1988) consisting of a mixture of health and social care professionals were convened. The facilitator explored how such skills might promote evidence-based practice (EBP) in day-to-day work. Would EBP help address and/or resolve some of the problems which the groups met regularly? Could an evidence-based approach encourage joint working? Finally, the groups were encouraged to express their own views on the barriers to joint working. All three facilitators received the same briefing notes, so that the same topics were discussed in all three groups.

A grounded theory approach to analysis of the raw data was taken (Creswell, 1998). Thus, fresh transcripts were read and each freestanding idea or independent contribution was annotated and identified as a theme. These themes were individually reviewed and drawn together into higher-order codes

which were denoted categories. These categories constituted the higher-order level of analysis from which the theory – grounded in the testimony of the individual themes – was postulated. This approach has a long tradition in qualitative research (Glaser & Strauss, 1967), but takes a more Glaserian approach (Glaser, 1992).

Results

The main categories derived from the emerging themes were entitled **evidence-based practice** and **working together**.

Evidence-based practice

In general, the whole idea of using evidence to inform practice was welcomed by all the groups, on the grounds that it could help manage resources. There was a consensus that money should be prioritised to encourage evidence-based practice and an expectation in some groups that such activity could increase costs and involve a large time commitment. All groups recognised the importance of key players being involved in this activity.

The data reveal widespread concerns in the groups about applying research evidence in general, despite their overall enthusiasm for the activity. There were two strands of thought here. One described the difficulty of applying national data to a specific locality, and the second the generic difficulty of applying population evidence from randomised controlled trials to individuals – *'every person is different'*. Some participants were more enthusiastic than others about using evidence. *'Clinical practice does change with really sound studies'*, one person argued. But applying research evidence can be tricky, cautioned another, for example where a large randomised controlled trial had selected patients who simply were not representative of the population seen regularly in routine practice. One particularly poignant intervention recognised the threat posed by evidence-based medicine: *'Do I really want to accept I've been doing something futile for 20 years?'*.

The groups spent some time describing how their own working practice was affected by the particular geographical characteristics of their localities, such as isolation or seasonal working. One participant summed up these themes thus:

> *'A lot of the links we have to make tend to be in [name of town], but a lot of resources are centralised – that actually is quite a barrier when it comes to working at a local level'.*

Thus described, the locality context appeared to have an impact not simply on participants' own work, but also on their enthusiasm for working together.

The groups agreed that restricted financing could pose problems, not just to working together but also within the professional groups separately. While evidence-based practice might produce quality work, *'it is all over-shadowed with the finance of it all'*.

None of the groups had any difficulty in identifying a range of problems which could benefit from joint working. Judging by the amount of data collected for each topic, care of the elderly came out easily as the key issue to tackle, in terms of rehabilitation, respite care and the mental health of the elderly. Dementia, falls, bed-blocking and the reason for hospital admissions were other topics the groups wanted to tackle in this area.

Working together

Each group separately and spontaneously identified the theoretical advantages of professionals from health and social care working together:

> *'it's a great idea just to be able to communicate – leaving aside the fact that there's yet another meeting and it's time that we have to give up'.*

The participants perceived an advantage in the team approach to sharing knowledge and tackling problems. *'I guess, what we've been talking about, professional groups working together... mmm... those issues are for me about relationships'*, said one participant.

Data which described barriers to working together were identified at three levels. At the first level, professional or operational difficulties were discussed. Beyond this, data at a second, deeper level described problems about the very nature of health care and social care; this level has been called metaphysical. And finally a philosophical level was identified, where data relating to (perceived) fundamental differences in the medical and social models of practice were collated.

Barriers to working together – professional level

The operational difficulty of convening multi-professional groups was described in a large number of contributions from all three groups.

> *'We never get the right people around the table.'*

Within this data set, general practitioners specifically and repeatedly came in for criticism for their failure to attend multidisciplinary groups. Some other barriers to the idea of working together were identified. These include divisions between health and education, which were described as being *'poles apart'*. Confusion about the roles and responsibilities within non-doctor professional groups was identified.

Barriers to working together – metaphysical level

A set of data was identified under the broad heading of working together which seemed to transcend mere day-to-day operational issues and dwelt upon the inherent nature of the problems faced by these professional groups, which in itself might render joint working difficult. Patients did not come describing literal, discrete and identified health or social care problems, but with diffuse, undifferentiated concerns. The groups recognised the difficulty general

research into practice

practitioners experience facing such 'undifferentiated problems', which they tend to see more than others because they are so accessible.

Within separate professions, some individuals recognised the changing nature of the demands on their professional group. *'I don't think I do what I was trained to do'*, commented one social worker. Some were simply *'so busy we can't do this job properly'*, while others cited the problems associated with rising expectations as chronically stressful.

Barriers to working together – philosophical level

Two of the groups recognised serious conceptual difficulties to working together based on a perceived dichotomy of approach between health and social care:

'the basis of the assessment is different, GPs think in terms of treatment'

'we've got the problem of them working most specifically with the social model as opposed to the medical model'.

The groups considered that there was at least the *'potential for argument from polarisation of views'* and included what they described as *'a huge variation in the GPs' practice of medicine'* as a potential impediment to working together.

All three groups explored perceived differences between the medical and social models of practice. The data are best illustrated by this extract.

'Medicine is much more easily definable.... with medication you either take it or you don't; with social services you are talking about people and there are an infinite variety of variables.'

This perceived difference in professional approach extended not only to the assessment of individual cases, but also to treatment decisions generally and to the application of research evidence.

Discussion

From these data, there appears to be a general willingness among these participants from health and social care to work together. They felt that it would improve relationships, improve practice and ultimately lead to better service provision. Adopting an evidence-based approach seemed compatible with collaboration; money should be diverted to encourage it. At the least it was another avenue for better communication. An evidence-based approach could help joint working by encouraging a joint approach to problem-solving, which in turn might lead to a joint improvement in IT skills, and maybe, as a consequence, better library facilities. But enthusiasm for an evidence-based approach was not unrestrained. At a personal level, there was the threat that the evidence would reveal that customary practice was ineffective (or worse), and at a methodological level, there was the problem of relating population research to individuals. These concerns have been rehearsed elsewhere, and standard educational strategies can be adopted in response to them (Daws, 1996).

As far as pitfalls to working together were concerned, the data show that there are concerns on a number of levels. Issues of finance and geography were strong themes. Evidence-based practice might increase costs, some thought, although this view has been rejected by the 'high priests' of evidence-based medicine (Sackett & Rosenburg, 1995).

At a much more profound level, the groups expressed two further sets of perceived barriers to working together. They related to the metaphysics of working together and philosophical differences in the way that the participants described the medical and social care approach to professional practice. Of all the themes which emerged in the analysis, these represent the most serious challenge for senior people in health and social care who want to encourage collaborative evidence-based practice.

Two lines of thinking emerged. On the one hand, the participants identified deeply distressing parts of their own work, like the inescapable personal unhappiness or insuperable disadvantage which many of the clients experienced. Here, the groups seemed to be saying that, despite a professional preparation for their work based on a professional analysis of the problem, many of the issues which presented to them were existential, insoluble and utterly dispiriting for the individuals involved. In itself, the groups were suggesting, this could diminish enthusiasm for evidence-based approaches and working together.

The second level of problems in this category may partly explain this. The participants from social care thought that there was a strong difference between their own philosophical attitude to practice and their ideas of how, at the same level, those in health care – particularly doctors – approached their work. There could be differences, for example, in the way that research was applied, they argued, depending on whether the social model or the medical model of practice was being applied. Medicine was perceived by those in social care to be much more definite, interventionist and standardised than social care. And this view was reciprocated by some of the general practitioners, who described the approach of social care workers as diffuse.

Importantly, the relationship between the two approaches was not seen as potentially complementary or symbiotic. Rather, the groups chose adversarial metaphors like 'the problem', 'argument' or 'polarisation' when discussing how the two approaches related to each other. And this distinction did not have simply an intellectual relevance; those in social care argued that the medical approach to service delivery could explain the variation in clinical medical practice that the social care professionals perceived in their locality. But what is also interesting about this set of data is the absence of any consideration of variation in

practice by other professionals in the groups, either social workers or nurses.

Future prospects

The results of this research fit with other reports on joint training (Hunter, 1993; Corney, 1995), and the authors acknowledge that the data do not demonstrate improved collaboration. We cannot assume, as Loxeley (1997) has warned, that skills from joint working will just emerge 'through a sort of osmosis' as professionals learn together about a specific topic.

While the operational problems to working together seemed predictable and relatively easy to respond to, the philosophical distinctions which appear to be firmly held by the participants in these groups do represent a substantial barrier to working together. There is a recognised theoretical basis in medicine on which this antithesis may be founded, reflecting either a traditional biomedical approach to clinical practice, or a more interpretative, contextual view of clinical work (Evans & Sweeney, 1998). Such a distinction could also be interpreted as a continuation of the ancient tension between the Hygeian and the Aesclepian traditions of medical practice. While the former seeks to ensure the inner and environmental equilibrium within a individual, the latter, which conventional medicine tends to embrace, sees an inherent disorder in sickness and seeks to bring measured external forces to bear to restore order (Greaves, 1996).

How can we tackle this? While the social services staff's concerns about the nature of medical practice are not new, it is curious that within medicine itself there is a vibrant debate about just how robust, scientific and black-and-white medicine is (Dixon & Sweeney, 2000). It is perhaps a lack of familiarity, then, which leads to these conflicting views. If each professional group understood more about how their

research into practice

colleagues worked, how they took decisions, the elusive and uncertain way in which many of these decisions had to be taken, there might be greater motivation to collaborate. Looking at existing evidence which is relevant to common problems faced might underpin this.

Within medicine, a working model exists which could address these issues. The Significant Event Audit (SEA) has been developed from industry and tailored to primary care (Pringle *et al*, 1995). It has gained in popularity within general practice and is now one of the compulsory criteria for a higher qualification of general practice (Fellowship by Assessment of the Royal College of General Practitioners). In SEA, a practice team meets, usually monthly, to address any issue regarded as significant by any member of the practice team. This could be a major clinical issue, for example how someone who collapsed in the surgery was managed, or an important managerial issue, like how to handle influenza vaccination of 1,000 at-risk individuals. But it is also a forum where a team can congratulate themselves, for example by discussing an improved repeat prescription service or reducing delays for patients seen by the nurse. Of course, it will be the forum where complaints will be aired and investigated, but the approach here is not judicial or blaming, rather what the practice can learn from and do about a particular complaint. Any staff member can bring an issue to the forum, confidentiality is stressed, minutes are recorded, and an audit of actions based on the decisions thus minuted is undertaken regularly.

Recent evidence for primary care suggests that SEA improves understanding of others' roles, assists team working, helps to develop basic problem-solving skills and encourages an .atmosphere of reflective practice (Westcott *et al*, 2000). To be successful, SEA needs good leadership, has to establish a non-judgmental atmosphere and should encourage equality of participation. Individuals should be nominated to carry out any decisions arising from a significant event audit, and these actions should be audited regularly too.

The data from this study suggest broad enthusiasm for an evidence-based approach to practice, and a willingness to prioritise it as a learning need. But collaboration means more than just sharing a model of good practice; it means talking together, reflecting and a willingness to understand how other professional groups in health care operate and improve. Significant Event Auditing has begun to achieve that for primary care teams. It is to be commended to social care, and should be developed as a joint effort. Maybe the key to the solution was best expressed by this participant:

'It's people who communicate, organisations don't communicate'.

References

Abramsom, J. S. & Mizrahi, T. (1996) When social workers and physicians collaborate: positive and negative inter-disciplinary experiences. *Social Work* **14** (3) 270–182.

Clarke, N. (2000) *Improving the Performance of Social Services.* PhD Thesis (pending). University of Exeter, Exeter.

Corney, R. (1995) Mental health services. In: P. Owens, J. Carier & J. Horder (Eds) *Interprofessional Issues in Community and Primary Health Care.* London: MacMillan.

Creswell, J. W. (1998) *Qualitative Enquiry and Research Design.* London: Sage Publications.

Dalley, B. (1991) Beliefs and behaviour: professionals and the policy process. *Journal of Ageing Studies* **5** (2) 163–180.

Daws, M. G. (1996) On the need for evidence-based general and family practice. *Evidence Based Medicine* **1** 68–69.

Department of Health/Social Services Inspectorate (1989) *Working with Child Sexual Abuse: Guidance for Training Social Services Staff.* London: HMSO.

Department of Health/Social Services Inspectorate (1991) *Care Management and Assessment: Managers' Guide.* London: HMSO.

research into practice

Dixon, M. & Sweeney, K. G. (2000) *The Human Effect in Medicine: Theory, Research and Practice.* Oxford: Radcliffe Press.

Evans, M. & Sweeney, K. G. (1998) *The Human Side of Medicine.* Occasional Paper 72. London: Royal College of General Practitioners.

Gambetta, D. (1998) *Trust: Making and Breaking Co-operative Relations.* Oxford: Blackwell.

Glaser, B. (1992) *Emergence Versus Forcing Basics of Grounded Theory Analysis.* California: The Sociology Press.

Glaser, B. & Strauss, A. (1967) *The Discovery of Grounded Theory.* Chicago: Aldine.

Greaves, D. (1996) *Mystery in Western Medicine.* Avebury Publishing: Aldershot.

Hunter, D. (1993) 'It's not the knowing, it's the doing'. *Health Service Journal* **21** October 7.

Leedham, I. & Wistow, G. (1992) *Community Care and General Practitioners.* Leeds: Nuffield Institute.

Loxeley, A. (1997) *Collaboration in Health and Welfare – Working with Difference.* London: Jessica King Publishers.

Morgan, D. L. (1988) *Focus Groups as Qualitative Research.* London: Sage Publications.

Pringle, M., Bradley, C. P., Carmichael, C. M., Wallace, H. & Moore, A. (1995) *Significant Event Audit.* Occasional Paper 70. Exeter: Royal College of General Practitioners.

Sackett, D. L. & Rosenburg, W. M. C. (1995) The need for evidence-based medicine. *Journal of the Royal Society of Medicine* **88** 620–624.

Sheldon, B. (1994) Biological and social factors in mental disorders: implications for services. *International Journal of Psychiatry* **40** (2) 87–105.

Westcott, R., Sweeney, G. & Stead, J. (2000) Significant Event Audit in practice: a preliminary study. *Family Practice* **17** (2) 173–179.

Correspondence to KGSweeney@exeter.ac.uk

Paper 2

Family Practice
© Oxford University Press 2000

Vol. 17, No. 5
Printed in Great Britain

A preliminary study of the decision-making process within general practice

Rebecca Mears and Kieran Sweeney[a]

Mears R and Sweeney K. A preliminary study of the decision-making process within general practice. *Family Practice* 2000; **17**: 428–429.

Objective. The aim of the present study was to explore the factors that contribute to the process of decision making within general practice, over and above evidence-based information.

Methods. A qualitative study was conducted using semi-structured interviews on a purposeful sample of GPs, based in the South West of England. Each interview was tape-recorded and transcribed verbatim.

Results. Five broad categories emerged from the data: practitioner; patient; practitioner–patient relationship; verbal and non-verbal communication; evidence-based medicine; and external factors.

Conclusion. The nature of general practice is such that the process of making clinical decisions is complex. In an era when GPs are being overwhelmed by evidence-based information, consideration needs to be given to the implications that the nature of the decision-making process has upon the way 'evidence' is constructed and promoted within general practice.

Keywords. Clinical decision making, decision making, evidence-based medicine, general practice, GP.

Introduction

Defined as the "conscientious, explicit and judicious use of current best evidence",[1] evidence-based medicine (EBM) has emerged as a new paradigm for medical practice. Awareness of the latest scientific evidence, the ability critically to appraise literature and assess the generalizability have been identified as integral to the practice of EBM. However, the evaluation of evidence within general practice is often illogical and irrational[2] and it cannot be assumed that GPs practise the principles underpinning EBM in their decision making.

The purpose of this study was to conduct a preliminary investigation of the factors that contribute to the clinical decision-making process within general practice, over and above the assumptions underlying evidence-based information.

Received 4 November 1999; Revised 6 April 2000; Accepted 16 May 2000.
Department of Epidemiology and Public Health, Institute of Child Health, Great Ormond Street Hospital, 30 Guilford Street, London WC1N 1EH and [a]Research Development Support Unit, Postgraduate Medical School, University of Exeter, Exeter, UK.

Methods

Semi-structured interviews were conducted using a 'convenient', purposeful sample of GPs, who were either based in a research-based general practice or involved in continuing medical education.

Data collection

RM conducted semi-structured interviews with each practitioner for ~1 hour. Each GP gave both their written and verbal consent. Interviews were audio-taped and transcribed verbatim and, to ensure reliability, each transcript was read independently by RM and another researcher who was blinded to the study aims. Their results were compared in order to establish a degree of congruence and disparity. A degree of congruence of 80% was deemed acceptable.[4] Respondent validation was also used to ensure that the data analysis and interpretation were an accurate reflection of the views of the practitioners.

Results and discussion

All five practitioners were based in practices within the South West of England. One of the practitioners was female. Their mean age was 47 years (range 40–54 years), and three of the practices were training practices.

The results indicated five broad categories that contribute to the decision-making process within general practice: practitioner; patient; practitioner–patient relationship; communication; EBM; and external factors.

Practitioner

All of the practitioners described that previous clinical experiences, and their own philosophy of health and clinical beliefs had an impact upon clinical decision making: "doctors also have their own philosophy of health, and there's no reason why they shouldn't . . ." (Interview 1), and "it's the things that go wrong that imprint on your memory . . ." (Interview 3).

Patient

Among all respondents, there was also recognition that understanding patients' cultural beliefs, background and attitudes is integral to the decision-making process: "you have to respect their beliefs and values . . ." (Interview 5), "you have to know where the patients are coming from . . . and what their beliefs are" (Interview 1).

Practitioner–patient relationship

Respondents all referred to the importance of maintaining good relations with patients: ". . . patients are technicolour and actually the relationship is technicolour" (Interview 1). One practitioner described a situation in which he had bowed to the expectations of the patient for the sake of maintaining good relations: "the nature of the relationship is one that continues and goes on and there may be far more important issues coming up than this trivial issue of whether or not you prescribe penicillin . . ." (Interview 1).

Verbal and non-verbal communication

All of the respondents mentioned being aware of the language that they used during a consultation: "you've got to pitch what you say at a level that the patient will understand . . ." (Interview 3). Two respondents cited non-verbal cues as informing the clinical decisions that they made, e.g. whether or not to prescribe: "patients do give quite strong messages without necessarily expressing them verbally, about what they want" (Interview 1).

Evidence-based medicine (EBM)

There was a pervading feeling among respondents that the EBM approach to clinical decision making did not allow for the complexities inherent within the decision-making process in general practice: "only a proportion of clinical decision making is ever to do with research . . ." (Interview 4), ". . . EBM measures the things that can be measured . . ." (Interview 2).

External factors

Time, cost and the media were three factors extraneous to the practitioner and patient most commonly cited as influencing the decision-making process: "GPs are conscious of society's views but particularly cost . . ." (Interview 3), "time is critical, we don't have very long, that's the problem" (Interview 5), ". . . the media are more powerful than anything else" (Interview 5).

Study limitations

Due to both time and financial constraints, the sample size in this study was very small. This factor represents a major limitation for this study; the results are therefore presented as preliminary.

Conclusion

The findings of this preliminary investigation suggest, in support of previous studies,[3,5] that the approach to clinical decision making within general practice is multifaceted. The complexities inherent within this process are not reflected in the 'linear' approach of formulating a clear clinical question, promoted within the EBM model.[1]

In an era when GPs are being overwhelmed by evidence-based information, consideration needs to be given to the implications that this has upon the way in which 'evidence' is constructed and presented to GPs. Any evidence-based model aimed at general practice needs to be compatible with its complex, and often irrational, illogical nature.

References

1 Sackett DL, Richardson WS, Rosenberg W, Haynes BR. *Evidence-based Medicine—How to Practice and Teach EBM*. Churchill Livingstone, 1997.
2 Sweeney K, MacAuley D, Pereira Gray D. Personal significance—the third dimension. *Lancet* 1998; **351**: 134–136.
3 Tomlin K, Humphrey C, Rogers S. General practitioners' perceptions of effective health care. *Br Med J* 1999; **318**: 1532–1535.
4 Miles MB, Huberman AM. *Qualitative Data Analysis*. 2nd edn. Thousand Oaks, CA: Sage, 1994.
5 Jacobson LD, Edwards AGK, Granier SK, Butler CC. Evidence-based medicine and general practice. *Br J Gen Pract*, 1997; **47**: 449–452.

Paper 3

Primary care

Why general practitioners do not implement evidence: qualitative study

A C Freeman, K Sweeney

Abstract

Objectives To explore the reasons why general practitioners do not always implement best evidence.
Design Qualitative study using Balint-style groups.
Setting Primary care.
Participants 19 general practitioners.
Main outcome measures Identifiable themes that indicate barriers to implementation.
Results Six main themes were identified that affected the implementation process: the personal and professional experiences of the general practitioners; the patient-doctor relationship; a perceived tension between primary and secondary care; general practitioners' feelings about their patients and the evidence; and logistical problems. Doctors are aware that their choice of words with patients can affect patients' decisions and whether evidence is implemented.
Conclusions General practitioner participants seem to act as a conduit within the consultation and regard clinical evidence as a square peg to fit in the round hole of the patient's life. The process of implementation is complex, fluid, and adaptive.

Introduction

Evidence based medicine is based on universally appealing ethical and clinical ideals in that it promotes the identification of the best methods of health care and helps patients and doctors to make better informed choices.[1] Its framework for searching out and critically appraising evidence helps doctors ask answerable questions to help patients make appropriate decisions.[2]

Although evidence based medicine has heightened awareness of the most effective management strategies for many conditions, much of the evidence is not acted on in everyday clinical practice.[3] Numerous strategies to improve implementation of such evidence have been tested,[4] and various impediments have been identified.[5] General practitioners have been cautious about the evidence based model generally.[6] In one study that asked general practitioners why they depart from evidence based practice, the commonest reason was reluctance to jeopardise their relationship with the patient.[7] Apparent hesitation in applying evidence in specific clinical areas such as atrial fibrillation has been attributed to patients' unwillingness to take the drugs.[8]

In a recent questionnaire study of general practitioners' attitudes to evidence based medicine, answers to an open question suggested that there are unique barriers to implementing evidence in general practice within a patient centred context.[9] This study set out to explore the issues raised by these responses. We used a qualitative approach to explore the reasons why and circumstances in which doctors had not implemented evidence they knew about.

Participants and methods

Three focus groups of established general practitioners were set up in three areas, each located around a different district general hospital. The hospitals were in the south west of England and covered the area served by a single primary care research network. Each area is geographically separate by about 80 km and tends to develop its own medical community. The groups did not contact each other throughout the study and were not in regular social or professional contact outside the study. By using these separate groups, we aimed to improve the trustworthiness of the data.

Participants were asked to discuss their behaviour in individual cases, which could be seen as sensitive. We therefore adapted the standard focus group techniques to use a Balint-style model. This style of group work is widely recognised in general practice, and derives from the work of the psychotherapist Michael Balint.[10] The focus groups were not pure Balint groups because they did not include a psychoanalyst. However, a widely used modified form of these original Balint groups has become common in general practice.[11] The particular Balint-style feature of these groups that distinguished them from standard focus groups was that each meeting focused around the case notes of a particular patient, the doctor-patient relationship, and the feelings that were generated. Basic rules of confidentiality are a prerequisite for convening the group, and the participants agree not to discuss material raised in the group outside. The same group of doctors met on several occasions in the hope that, as the group matured, they would feel more comfortable about exploring honest reasons behind their failure to implement evidence.

The groups consisted of six to eight volunteer general practitioners, each led by an experienced group leader. The group leader was given an honorarium to lead and administer the groups and operate the tape

Somerset and North and East Devon Primary Care Research Network, Institute of General Practice, School of Postgraduate Medicine and Health Sciences, Exeter EX2 5DW
A C Freeman
general practice research facilitator
K Sweeney
general practice research facilitator

Correspondence to:
A C Freeman
PCRN@exeter.ac.uk

BMJ 2001;323:1–5

recorder. The plan was to have the groups meet about once a month on six occasions, each meeting lasting about two hours. Two of the groups consisted of doctors from different practices and one group comprised doctors from one practice. Participating doctors represented a mix of urban, rural, and semirural practices. There were a total of 19 doctors: 13 men and six women. Their length of time as a principal varied from three to 25 years. Fourteen held the membership examination of the Royal College of General Practitioners, and seven were general practice trainers.

At each meeting, a group member was asked to present the details of a case in which he or she had knowingly not followed evidence based practice. Participants were advised to anonymise the patient details and not present any material that could lead to the identification of a particular patient. We asked the groups to discuss the case and explore the implementation issues arising from it as well as the doctor's feelings about these issues. The local research ethics committee approved the study.

The researchers were not part of the group, but before the first meeting of each group a researcher attended and explained the research agenda. We explained that the individual doctors would be anonymous. We had no further contact with the groups. We returned copies of the transcripts to the groups, and each member understood that if they were not happy with the content that transcript would not be used.

The meetings were taped, and the tapes delivered to us. The tapes were transcribed, and each researcher separately analysed the transcripts. Each researcher used a grounded theory approach in developing theoretical principles (or at least explanatory principles).[12] This was to ensure that the coding of themes consistently and robustly followed grounded theory rules and that all the emerging themes were directly supported by verbatim data from the meetings. We did not set out with the overarching aim of generating theory from the findings.

We met to compare analysis and identify common themes. To ensure compatibility of analysis, we each analysed three transcripts jointly and the others separately. For the separate analyses, we were given the transcripts recorded out of our own area to minimise the recognition of names, accents, or circumstances that could lead to the identification of patients or participating doctors.

Results

Transcripts for 11 meetings were available for analysis. Two of the groups met six times each, and the third once only—that is, 13 meetings. The recordings of two of the groups could not be used because of poor sound quality.

The main clinical areas the general practitioners discussed included hypertension, ischaemic heart disease, and anticoagulation. Other topics developed in the groups discussion included diabetes, chronic obstructive pulmonary disease, menorrhagia, cholesterol, and the use of investigations. Six main themes emerged from the data (box).

> **Main themes from data**
>
> The process of implementing clinical evidence is affected by the personal and professional experiences of the doctor
>
> The relationship that the doctor has with individual patients also affects the process
>
> There is a perceived tension between primary and secondary care: the doctors thought that specialists approach evidence based practice differently
>
> The practitioner's feelings about their relationships with patients and about the evidence have an important role in modifying how clinical evidence is applied
>
> The doctor's choice of words in consultations can sway patients to accept or reject clinical evidence. Doctors realise this and can use it to pre-empt patients' decisions
>
> Implementation comes up against logistical problems, which affect how evidence is applied

Personal and professional experience of practitioner

Our data show that doctors' personal and professional experiences influence how clinical evidence is implemented. Despite being a relatively homogeneous group, the general practitioners' enthusiasm for the evidence and the way in which they implemented it varied. This seemed to be partly explained by their previous experience of clinical practice.

Two influences were relevant: the doctors' life experience and experience of hospital medicine as students or juniors doctors. "My grandfather died when he was shocked," recalled one participant, discussing anticoagulation in atrial fibrillation, "so I reach for a decent dose of warfarin and digoxin no hesitation at all." Another said: "I actually had two 50 year olds who had strokes from atrial fibrillation because they didn't get warfarin … that really hit me." In another group, one general practitioner said, " I lost a patient as an SHO, so that puts me off warfarin."

Accidents, mishaps, or spectacular clinical successes have a direct influence on subsequent practice. Commenting again on anticoagulation in atrial fibrillation, a participant exclaimed, "I'm back on it." This doctor had previously been uneasy about anticoagulating patients in atrial fibrillation but had recently seen one of his patients who was not given warfarin have a cerebrovascular event. This theme was taken up in another group: "But I suppose if we had a run of people who … then had terrible hemiplegias and ended up being a huge workload on the community … if we saw the ones the papers were talking about, we would probably be warfarin zealots, wouldn't we." One doctor summed up this view. thus: "We are influenced at least as much, if not more, by the experiences of individual patients as we are by the evidence."

Doctor's relationship with individual patients

Implementation was influenced by the relationships that doctors developed with their patients. "Even if the evidence was extremely good," one general practitioner said, "most of us would only ever interpret it in the context of the patient." Perceived patient characteristics could have a positive or negative effect on implementation. "Of course, if they're the sort who always want the specialist, then you follow their [the specialist's] advice." Another explained, " I think you have to judge how people feel about it. I try to get patients to reveal to me where they lie in the game ... from I want it mate to I don't want to know nothing about it doc ... I make tremendous judgments."

Patients could influence clinical decisions as a result of their own experiences. "Well he's a farmer, so every time he calls the vet he gets antibiotics." Another patient reportedly said, "My brother died on warfarin, I'm not taking rat poison." Some doctors found that personal relationships tended to make practising evidence based medicine "harder because you have a close relationship with them." At other times patients could simply block a doctor's attempts to practise evidence based medicine: "Sod that, says the patient, I'm fine."

The assumptions doctors made about their patients seemed at times paternalistic. Some were described by their doctor as " the type who did not want to rock the boat," others as "depressive cum fatalist." "Somatisers," declared one doctor, "eventually get something." By using these descriptions, the contributors were suggesting that their view of the patient modified how and when they applied the evidence.

One doctor built up the relationship with the patient by initially not following the guidelines and then, in a position of greater trust, was able to implement the guidelines properly. "I have now followed the guidelines of course, but in a sneaky way and it's taken about three months to do it."

Perceived tension between primary and secondary care

The general practitioners talked at length about their relationships with secondary care doctors. They felt that specialists approached evidence based practice differently, treating "diseases rather than patients" in a context that they perceived as much more controlled than the "real life" of general practice. On the whole, the relationship was described in pejorative terms. "They do seem a slightly different breed," one general practitioner said, referring to cardiologists. A doctor in another group described cardiologists as "being a bit of an evidence based mafia."

Specialists were accused of failing to realise just how tricky it was controlling some common diseases. "You get stroppy letters from the clinic saying your patient's blood pressure is still 160, and I go ... yes, yes, I know. You feel under pressure from the guidelines, but you know it's not from want of trying." In one group, quite a fundamental difference in approach to clinical practice between primary and secondary care was described. "A few hypertensives, without any symptoms, they're well. They're just running a risk. We give them a drug and a side effect—change the quality of their life," said one doctor. A female participant in the same group agreed, saying, "Show me one GP who doesn't think like this, show me one cardiologist who does. I mean, this is the problem, isn't it?"

Clinical evidence can evoke feelings among doctors and patients

For the doctors in our study, clinical evidence is not just an intellectually celibate commodity that is lifted out of medical journals and transferred to a patient. It has an emotional impact on practitioners and patients. "Yes it does make me feel anxious ... all the *BMJ*s, all the rags ... these people must be on warfarin." "With me mess-

ing about with his medication and trying to practise evidence based medicine, I found it was making him [the patient] feel more anxious." Sometimes the knowledge that the evidence existed, waiting to be applied, was seen as a burden in itself: "We get bogged down with perhaps putting the evidence first and consecrating it."

Another aspect of this theme reflected the doctors' feelings about the consequences of failing to act on clinical evidence. One participant poignantly described how, after the death of a young man who had been inadequately anticoagulated for a venous thrombosis, he felt unease "standing behind his widow in the greengrocer queue." Another group, taking up this theme, distinguished between probability and certainty, reflecting the tension general practitioners feel about predicting the clinical course in any one person: "You don't know, do you? You just don't know."

The group discussions also produced data that indicated doctors' familiarity with the evidence and a positive attitude to it. They described its importance to everyday practice: "I think it's always the basis for most of what I do ... it's fundamentally evidence based but it's tailored completely." They recognised that evidence based medicine gives new emphasis: "That is the one that I have been hammering, the diabetic blood pressures, to try and get them to 140/80, and I am certainly getting them better than I was but it is hard work." For some of the general practitioners evidence based medicine was revolutionary: "I think that is the first time I have become aware of one study, or group of studies, that has actually changed my practice within a week."

Words used by doctors can influence patients' decisions

Doctors realised that the words they chose to present the evidence could have a strong influence on the patient's decision. They effectively limited the options while seeming to invite the patient to make the decision. The contributors framed these themes with phrases such as "It's how you put it over," and "It depends on how you feed information to people." The semantics then affect the way in which evidence is implemented by swaying the patient in a particular direction. "There is a reasonable chance of you having a stroke in the next year or so if you don't do something about your blood pressure ... I'm as barbaric as that," commented one participant.

The participants realised that this in effect "pre-empted" the decision that they were encouraging patients to take during consultations. Some talked of "selling" a particular view on clinical evidence. This tension between encouraging autonomy and effectively limiting options by the slanted presentation of relevant material was a relatively strong theme: "I make these judgments in theory with the patient but probably on my own." Another contributor described the problem as, "How much are we obliged to persuade people, or do we let them make up their own minds?"

The choice of words or the use of metaphors like "slanting" or "selling" were mechanisms the doctors used to influence patients to make a decision about their treatment that was consistent with what the doctor had decided was appropriate. Doctors would refer to "rat poison" when describing warfarin if they felt its use would be difficult or inappropriate, or describe pills as "having been shown to keep the heart young" when they wanted a patient to agree to treatment. When a doctor argued that it "depends on how you feed information to people," other members of the focus groups debated the issue hotly: doctors might influence decisions, they said, but patients can refuse to accept advice too.

Logistics of general practice

The doctors in this study described some tricky logistical problems that made them less enthusiastic about implementing clinical evidence. "Risky," "hard work," and a "hassle" both for doctors and patients were typical descriptions of the problems of starting treatment. One doctor said, "The problem is starting him on the ACE because he is very anxious about any medication change, and every time you change the medication it entails another four or five visits to go and see him and to try and reassure him that he is on the right medication."

Complications always tended to happen "over the weekend," and those practitioners who, for example, did not always have nursing staff to help do blood tests seemed to be less enthusiastic about implementing evidence on anticoagulation. When discussing the potential side effects of warfarin, one participant said, " It's not a minor bleed if your patient is 30 miles from the nearest transfusion service."

Knowing the patient's personal situation influenced implementation too. Doctors took into account the patient's behaviour, capabilities, or rural location when making decisions. One doctor felt reluctant to anticoagulate one 88 year old woman because "she had an alcohol problem, kept falling. She was forever in casualty being stitched up, bandaged up, whatever."

Discussion

This study suggests that the general practitioner acts as a conduit in consultations in which clinical evidence is one commodity. For some doctors the evidence had clarified practice, focused clinical effort, and sometimes radically altered practice. But a stronger theme from our data is that doctors are shaping the square peg of the evidence to fit the round hole of the patient's life. The nature of the conduit is determined partly by the doctors' previous experiences and feelings. These feelings can be about the patient, the evidence itself, or where the evidence has come from (the hospital setting). The conduit is also influenced by the doctor-patient relationship. The precise words used by practitioners in their role as conduit can affect how evidence is implemented. In some settings, logistical problems will diminish the effectiveness of the conduit.

Strengths

The strengths of our study derive from the fact that three groups were held separately (enhancing the trustworthiness of identified themes). There was good concordance in the analysis of jointly reviewed transcripts, and validation by respondents did not show serious disagreement with the analysis. One group could not continue in the study, and dropped out. This group consisted of doctors in a single practice; one of the partners was enthusiastic about the project but was

What is already known on this topic
General practitioners do not always act on evidence in clinical practice
General practitioners are reluctant to jeopardise their relationship with the patient and sometimes feel that patients are unwilling to take drugs

What this study adds
Implementation of evidence by general practitioners is a complex and fluid process
Decisions are influenced by the doctor's personal and professional experience as well as by their knowledge of and relationship with the patient
Doctors' choice of words can influence patients' decisions about treatment

unable to sustain the other partners' interest. Because the group consisted of doctors in a single practice, the discussions involved the whole practice allocating time whereas in the other groups, individual general practitioners made their own arrangements to attend.

For the two groups that met six times, the Balint format seemed to work well. The doctors spoke honestly about difficult clinical situations in which their practice was incompatible with the principles of evidence based medicine. Over the course of the meetings, doctors developed sufficient confidence in the confidentiality of the group to allow them to speak in a way that probably could not have been captured as well by another qualitative instrument. Semistructured interviews might have offered an alternative: but careful listening to these tapes suggests that the honest interaction among group members encouraged individuals to be more explicit about their experiences than they might have been in a one to one interview.

Implementation of evidence

Doctors in the groups were talking about situations in which they already knew the evidence but had not implemented it. Although the groups did not confine their discussion exclusively to incidents in which the clinical evidence was not applied, the data focus wholly on implementation issues. We felt that if a wider brief had been given to the groups—for example, to discuss implementation generally—the detail of the difficulties these practitioners had implementing evidence would have been less likely to come up. There was plenty of evidence that the doctors were implementing evidence and were happy to do so. The data also indicated that doctors were working together with patients and for the benefit of their patients. Sometimes these factors and the doctor's experience lead to the conclusion that strictly sticking to the rules of guidelines is not appropriate. Whether that is the strength of individual doctoring in a long standing and trusting relationship with a patient or a weakness remains open to debate.

The doctors associated evidence based medicine with randomised controlled trials and systematic reviews. There was no data to show that they were aware of evidence from qualitative or observational research, although such studies are beginning to inform evidence based medicine.

Primary care

Put together, these themes illustrate the complexity of implementing evidence from well structured clinical trials in individual patients. Our findings are supported by other studies in the United Kingdom,[8][13] the Netherlands,[7] and Australia.[14] In some ways, our study illustrates what Kernick has described as the parallel universes of scientific research and general practice.[15] We argue that the doctors in this study were exploring personal importance—that is, the "key to the transfer of an idea to and the evaluation and interpretation of an idea by the doctor and patient together."[16] Evidence is not implemented in a simple linear way, as some definitions of evidence based practice imply, but in an evolving process whereby reciprocal contributions from the doctor and the patient over time influence how evidence ultimately is used.

We thank the general practitioners who gave their time to help in this research.

Contributors: ACF conceived the idea for this project, was involved at every stage of the study, and contributed to the analysis and all sections of the final paper. KS was involved at all stages of the study, and contributed to the analysis and all sections of the final paper. ACF is the guarantor.

Funding: This research was supported by a grant from the NHS South West Research and Development Executive.

Competing interests: None declared.

1 Kerridge I, Lowe M, Henry D. Ethics and evidence based medicine. *BMJ* 1998;316:1151-3.

2 Strauss SE, Sackett DL. Using research findings in clinical practice. *BMJ* 1998;317:339-42.

3 Haynes RB, Sackett D, Guyatt G, Cook D. Transferring evidence from research to practice: overcoming barriers to application. *Evidenced-Based Medicine* 1997;2:68-9.

4 Oxman AD, Thomson MA, Davis DA, Haynes RB. No magic bullets: a systematic review of 102 trials of interventions to improve professional practice. *Can Med Assoc J* 1995;153:1423-31.

5 Budd J, Dawson S. *Influencing clinical practice: implementation of research and development results.* London: Management School, Imperial College of Science Technology and Medicine, 1994. (Report to North Thames Regional Health Authority.)

6 Sweeney KG. Evidence an uncertainty. In: Marinker M, ed. *Sense and sensibility in health care.* London: BMJ Publishing, 1996:59-87.

7 Veldhuis M, Wigersma L, Okkes I. Deliberate departures from good general practice: a study of motives among Dutch general practitioners. *Br J Gen Pract* 1998;48:1833-6.

8 Howitt A, Armstrong D. Implementing evidence based medicine in general practice: audit and qualitative study of antithrombotic treatment for atrial fibrillation. *BMJ* 1999;318:1324-7.

9 McColl A, Smith H, White P, Field J. General practitioner's perceptions of the route to evidence based medicine: a questionnaire survey. *BMJ* 1998;316:361-5.

10 Balint M. *The doctor, his patient and the illness.* London: Pitman, 1957.

11 Salinsky J. Psychoanalysis and general practice: what did the Romans do for us? *Br J Gen Pract* 2001;51:506.

12 Glaser B, Strauss A. *The discovery of grounded theory.* Chicago: Aldine, 1957.

13 Tomlin Z, Humphrey C, Rogers S. General practitioners' perceptions of effective health care. *BMJ* 1999;318:1532-5.

14 Mayer J, Piterman L. The attitudes of Australian GPs to evidence-based medicine: a focus group study. *Fam Pract* 1999;16:627-32.

15 Kernick DP. Muddling through in a parallel track universe [letter]. *Br J Gen Pract* 2000;50:325.

16 Sweeney KG, MacAuley D, Gray DP. Personal significance: the third dimension. *Lancet* 1998;351:134-6.

(Accepted 6 August 2001)

Paper 4

J Med Ethics: Medical Humanities 2001;27:20–25

A comparison of professionals' and patients' understanding of asthma: evidence of emerging dualities?

K G Sweeney, Karen Edwards, Jonathan Stead and David Halpin *University of Exeter and North and East Devon Health Authority*

Abstract

Despite an increase in the provision of services to patients with asthma, morbidity from the disease remains high. Recent research (outside asthma) has raised the possibility that patients may develop a conceptualisation of illnesses which is not entirely compatible with the prevailing biomedical view. This paper compares the way in which health care professionals and patients with asthma described various aspects of the illness, using an approach which considered the type of knowledge which might be used to construct the respective conceptualisations of asthma. A qualitative method is employed, using focus groups. Eight focus groups were convened, four of professionals and four of patients with asthma. Following the initial data analysis, the results were reviewed linguistically, with particular attention to the use of metaphor.

The health care professionals and patients participating in this study agreed broadly in their explanations of the aetiology and drug treatment of asthma. The data suggest lack of congruence in the development of treatment strategies and locus of control. Health care professionals and patients in this study used linguistically different metaphors to represent the disease: the former more frequently used metaphors evoking on-going processes, the latter visualising the chest (in their use of metaphor) as a static container, emptying and filling throughout the course of the disease. Two commentaries from philosophical and anthropological literature are considered in order to offer theoretical accounts relevant to this interpretation. The data suggest an emerging duality in the approach to treatment plans, in the roles played by professionals and patients with asthma, and in the different types of knowledge used by professionals and patients to construct their respective working models of asthma.

(J Med Ethics: Medical Humanities 2001;27:20–25)

Keywords: Asthma; metaphor; types of knowledge; epistemology; language

Introduction

Asthma is a common disease. Its prevalence is increasing, and despite a clearer understanding of its pathogenesis, morbidity and mortality from the disease remain high.[1-3] Most patients with asthma receive their care in the community, where a large number of general practices have responded by providing an increasing number of clinics, often led by specialist practice nurses.[4,5]

Despite this increase in service provision, recent surveys have shown that about half of all asthmatics continue to have night symptoms, and of that group, about half have such symptoms most nights.[4] There is no good indicator which can accurately predict adverse outcome in asthma.[6-8] Neither the peak expiratory flow rate (PEFR), symptom scores used in isolation, nor amount of bronchodilator use has been validated as a reliable predictor of outcome.[9,10]

Thus, the situation is paradoxical: health service provision for asthmatic patients is greater, and effective treatments are available, but morbidity from the disease remains high. A number of factors might contribute to this situation. There is published evidence which suggests low levels of adherence to seemingly logical, rational medical advice, particularly about the prophylactic use of steroids, and considerable dissonance between their recommended and actual use.[11] A person's attitude to and beliefs about asthma can influence the way treatments are used.[12] Thirdly, there could be misunderstandings between the doctor or nurse and patient about the nature of asthma or its treatment. A small number of semantic studies have shown how such potentially important differences in conceptualisation might be revealed by the vocabulary used by patients[13] or by their use of metaphor.[14-16] Beate *et al* have argued[17] that such dissonance might better be understood by considering theories of knowledge, citing Piaget's distinction between operational and figurative knowledge.[18,19] The dual taxonomy of knowledge alluded to by Piaget is echoed elsewhere, notably in Toulmin's separation of universal (essentially scientific) and existential (effectively personal, lived) knowledge.[20] Michael Polanyi's seminal text, *Personal Knowledge*, deals centrally with the distinction, arguing for a reconciliation between the two epistemologies.[21]

In a consultation about asthma or any other condition, the way in which information is packaged, expressed and exchanged is central. Such information, expressed in words, reflects the speaker's thinking and, in turn, knowledge base. Analysing consultations from this perspective, that is seeking to elicit the knowledge base which constitutes the bedrock of the exchange might, therefore, shed some light on how the participants think. Are the knowledge bases of the participants in such a consultation the same? If they are different, how can we elicit this, and what difference might that make?

This study set out to explore and compare how doctors and nurses on the one hand, and individuals with asthma on the other, expressed their understanding of various aspects of asthma. We attempted to compare the explanatory constructs of the two groups, to see if these would cast any light upon their respective understanding of how the disease worked, and to see if they influenced the way asthma was managed.

Methods

This paper reports on part of a large quantitative study of asthma, whose aim is to identify predictors of deterioration of asthma. In an introductory part of this study, the initial aim was to seek out and compare patient- and professional-based outcomes of asthma. Both sets of outcomes were then to be identified by analysing focus group data, with two series of focus groups (patient and professional) running in parallel. Focus groups were chosen as the preferred qualitative method because they were considered most likely to give rich data, particularly from patients, by allowing the group interaction to encourage the formation of patient-sensitive outcomes.[22] After the first two groups, however, it was obvious that little data about outcomes was emerging from the patient group, while the professionals very quickly rehearsed the well-known "medical" outcomes for the disease. Preliminary field notes of these meetings commented on the vocabulary used by some patients to describe the experience of having asthma, and noted how this contrasted with the conventional biomedical description of the professionals.

The research question therefore changed, in keeping with the heuristic nature of qualitative research.[23] The inquiry then focused on the precise way in which the two sets of participants described various aspects of asthma: the analysis centred on the use of language in their testimony. The research questions became: "Do patients and professionals describe asthma in different ways?"and "What can be inferred from this data about the knowledge base upon which these expressions are constructed?"

The study was convened in the South West of England, with approval from the local ethical committee. Two sets of focus groups were convened in parallel, four comprising professionals (doctors and nurses), and four drawn from patients with asthma. The professional groups comprised one separate group each of specialist doctors, secondary care nurses, general practitioners and practice nurses. Individuals with asthma were identified from general practice disease registers. To obtain a sufficient spread of patients with the type of asthma seen routinely in general practice, the sampling frame was stratified by age, and use of inhaled steroids (which was used as a proxy indication of asthma severity). The age bands were 16–44, and

45–65. Inhaler use was dichotomised as regular (defined as receiving a prescription for a steroid inhaler monthly over a period of twelve months) or infrequent (fewer received steroid inhaler prescriptions). Thus, one group each of young citizens who had received regular or infrequent steroid inhalers was convened, alongside two similar groups of older patients. None of the participants had experienced a hospital admission for asthma within the preceding year.

The groups, lasting 60–90 minutes, were convened between October 1997 and April 1998 according to published guidelines[24 25] and were facilitated by a researcher with experience of qualitative research.[26] The following questions were explored in each group: What is asthma? What are the treatments of asthma and how do they work/what do they do? What is it like to have asthma, or what must it be like? What are good outcomes of asthma treatment?

Data in the focus groups were recorded by audiotape with additional hand-written notes constituting a contact summary. A two-stage analysis was used. Firstly, a content analysis elicited the frequency with which terms were used in the participants' descriptions. Then a second-stage analysis identified the key conceptual themes in the data, linking them together in categories where appropriate. Once these categories had been completed, the researchers considered what type of knowledge might have been used in their construction, and also any power relationships suggested by their comparison. The trustworthiness of the coding frames was strengthened by review of an unmarked transcript by two experienced qualitative researchers and by presentation of the initial analysis to participants, who offered their comments on the analysis. Once the data analysis was completed, the initial findings were reviewed by one author (KE), an academic literary scholar, who commented specifically on the use of metaphor.

Results

COMPOSITION OF THE FOCUS GROUPS

Two nurse groups were convened, each consisting of six participants. All the general practice nurses participated in the shared care of asthma. The two doctor groups consisted of seven specialists, ranging from registrar to consultant, and five general practitioners, all of whom were trainers. Between four and seven participants attended each patient focus group. In total twenty-two participants attended the patient groups, nine of whom were men. The age range was 16–44, and 45–65 years. In all the groups, the participants were Caucasian and English-speaking.

Data analysis

WHAT IS ASTHMA?

In the professional groups, the term "inflammation" occurred more frequently than any other term and incorporated the notions of "swelling", "oedema" and "obstruction". Less frequently used terms were "narrow", "constrict", "smaller" and "tight". The doctors' groups described a detailed pathophysiological pathway for asthma which included descriptions of "leukotrienes" and "cytokines". One hospital doctor said: "I mean potentially it involves probably formal components of your inflammatory pathway, so probably certain parts can be switched off ... some are more prominent than others" (hospital doctor).

For the patients, the terms "constrict", "narrow" and "tight" predominate as descriptors of asthma. "Inflammation" was used less frequently and only once in the group of younger asthmatics using regular inhalers. The descriptions of asthma in these groups tended to be less conventionally biomedical, but obviously made sense to the participants, none of whom were challenged or derided for having idiosyncratic visions of what asthma was. One participant, for example said: "It seems more tight here just above my lungs, and someone's clenching them. This sounds ridiculous but it feels as if there's a load of carpet in them". (younger group, male, regular use of inhalers)

The dominant metaphor in the professional data in this section was of processes, for example "show pictures of swollen airway" (specialist nurse), or in the use of the phrase "path way . . . so probably certain parts can be switched off". For the patients the dominant metaphor was of containers : "It's like a windsock" (younger, infrequent use) "Hubbly bubbly pipes," (younger, frequent use).

WHAT ARE THE TREATMENTS FOR ASTHMA AND HOW DO THEY WORK?

The professional groups identified beta stimulant drugs and corticosteroids as the essential drugs for treating asthma. As one specialist nurse said: "one opens up the airway, the other stops it closing". The professional groups stressed the prospective benefits of using corticosteroids: "one makes you better at the time, the other keeps you better for tomorrow" (general practitioner). Thus, treatment strategies could or should be planned prospectively. The professional groups saw steroids as central to disease control, but recognised that patients were sometimes apprehensive about using them: "They're [patients] worried when you say this is a steroid inhaler and you give quite a little spiel about this being quite safe" (general practitioner). Sometimes patients did not fully "understand" their role. Consider this exchange:

(Nurse speaker 3): "It's quite interesting, they don't seem to be aware of the significance of their preventer, like you say."

(Nurse speaker 4) "It's because they didn't think they needed it."

(Nurse speaker 3) "Yes, that's the commonest thing."

The patients' groups identified salbutamol and beclomethasone as the two main treatments. The patients referred to these by their brand names (Ventolin and Becotide respectively) and these brand names appear in the patients' remarks reported here. There was a clear consensus about the effect of Ventolin: "The quickest relief. Less than a minute. Straight away" (older female infrequent use). The role of Becotide was less clear. "It's a medication which soothes" (young female, frequent use). "In the theory, I believe, I think it coats your lungs" (younger male, frequent use).

The patient groups confirmed the professionals' concerns about apprehension and understanding of steroids. Fear of the use of steroid inhalers was repeatedly described by the patients, who linked the use of Becotide with suppression of disease activity and with a decreased need for regular Ventolin use. The intermittent use of Becotide was a clear theme: "I only take Becotide when I've got something happening I can't possibly miss" (younger female, regular inhaler use). Often, an individual's decision to use Becotide was based upon a previous experience of it, (and not, as the professionals might have hoped, on its therapeutic rationale). "I take it if I get bad or get a cold ... on to my browns three or four days then it works. All the bad stuff comes towards it and bounces off it or gets eaten possibly. Maybe absorbed" (younger male, frequent inhaler use). This sometimes led individuals to act against medical advice to use Becotide continuously. "When you haven't got a tight chest you haven't got asthma, I just forget to take Becotide" (older group, male, infrequent inhaler use). Here, the participants seem to be constructing treatment plans retrospectively, based upon their accumulated experience of asthma.

THE EXPERIENCE OF ASTHMA: WHAT IS IT (OR MUST IT BE) LIKE?

Both the professionals and the patients agreed that asthma was a stigma which could cause embarrassment and restrictions in sporting, and some social, activities. This led some patients, in the view of the professionals, to resist the diagnosis: "They're not prepared to play the sick role, they deny the diagnosis." (general practitioner) Teenagers were more likely to do this, perhaps because, "they have no sense of their own mortality do they?" (community nurse). Asthma could be frightening, embarrassing and impair social activities, the professionals suggested.

The patients' data produced some poignant descriptions of the stigma and embarrassment attached (in their view) to having asthma. Sometimes, patients felt they should use their inhalers out of sight. "I'd sneak out on me *(sic)* own to use my inhalers so nobody could see it." (older male, infrequent use of inhaler) "I go to the loo" [to use inhalers] (younger male, frequent inhaler use). One individual reported: "Asthmatics at school were wimps. I don't want to be thought of as an invalid," (older male, infrequent inhaler use).

HOW DO YOU MANAGE (YOUR) ASTHMA?

Within the professionals' data, a clear responsibility for educating patients about asthma emerged, with nurses seen as key players. Within this educational

Table 1

Theme	Professional group	Patient group
What is asthma? Content analysis, main descriptors	"Inflammation", "swelling", "oedema", "obstruction"	"Constrict", "narrow", "tight"
Dominant metaphor	Process	Container
Treatment perspective	Prospective	Retrospective
Managing asthma	Prior professional responsibility assumed, and then transferred	Patient as experts : "I know my asthma better than anybody"
Locus of control	Operational (Piaget)	Figurative (Piaget)
Taxonomy of knowledge used in constructing the model of asthma	Universal (Toulmin)	Existential (Toulmin)

theme, the nurses described a relationship between professionals and patients which most closely resembled a teacher-pupil relationship. For example, when one professional commented on some patients refusing "to go to classes", (community nurse) the contact summary confirmed a group consensus. Within this teacher-pupil relationship, the professional groups perceived the need to keep clinical messages "simple": "I don't mean to be rude, but I mean you need to make it as basic as possible," (specialist nurse).

In one of the early patient groups an individual spontaneously reported: "I think you can generally advise yourself... . I think I can advise myself better."(younger male, frequent inhaler use). The facilitator tested this piece of testimony on that group and subsequent groups, and the contact summary confirms that there was a strong feeling among the individuals that they were experts in their own disease. "I know my asthma better than anybody." (older female, frequent inhaler use). This data evokes a tension in roles: the professionals with their desire to act as teachers, and the patients' sometimes distressing descriptions of their own expertise.

A subsidiary theme within this category suggested that patients may be the victims of their own actions. "Some have really brought it upon themselves because they smoke," (practice nurse). Referring to patients whose asthma was poorly controlled one practice nurse commented: "you have allowed it to take over." Many of the participants agreed that their asthma was not always well controlled. Some blamed themselves when they experienced exacerbations of asthma "I feel guilty getting bad and having to go to the doctor quick—to get a nebuliser—you know. I hang on and hang on." (younger female, infrequent inhaler use). The concept of guilt associated with exacerbations was vivid, for example, when the deterioration occurred at a friend's house thus causing inconvenience). Some admitted not wanting to interrupt their normal planned activities, or assumed that the deterioration they were experiencing would be transitory.

By contrast, discussion of the locus of control in asthma by the professional group suggested prior ownership of responsibility for the disease by the professional before returning or yielding it back to the patient. "We have to put control onto the person themselves (*sic*) to manage it," commented one practice nurse, a proposition which could be tricky with "difficult patients, where you have to allow them to take responsibility".

WHAT DO YOU THINK ARE GOOD OUTCOME MEASURES FOR THE TREATMENT OF ASTHMA?
The specialist groups easily rehearsed the conventional outcome measures for asthma: absence of wheeze, absence of cough, absence of early morning waking, ability to perform exercise, and not having to take time off work.

The patient groups did not specifically identify these conventional outcome measures in detail. Rather, they reported that they did not want to be embarrassed or fearful of their asthma, nor inconvenienced by it. "I want a totally normal life" (younger female, infrequent inhaler use), said one group member. "Just not to have to use inhalers," (younger male, infrequent inhaler use) commented another. On the whole, individuals in these citizen groups felt they could sense any deterioration in symptoms themselves. Little was added to that impression by recording the peak flow rate. "I only do peak flow rate to see the nurse or the doctor." (older participant, frequent use of inhaler).

We summarise the main points from these results in table 1.

Discussion
There are a number of drawbacks to this study. Firstly, focus groups, while appropriate initially, when differences in outcome were being explored, are probably not the best way to elicit differences in the use of language. We accept this, but argue that within these focus group, the patients were able to put forward ideas in their own words which the group could evaluate—for example by criticising a particularly peculiar vision of asthma. The field notes bear this out: the focus groups actually were "permission-giving" fora in which participants felt free to offer their private views when they saw that others were willing so to do. Secondly, the participants in these citizen groups could all be said to have accepted their diagnosis: Adams *et al* have written about the important group of asthmatics who deny their disease.[27] One could speculate that different data might have emerged from groups of such participants. Finally, no particular themes emerged to distinguish the understanding of asthma as a function either of age or inhaler use, the two strata upon which the groups were convened. However, several key ideas which emerged from our

data fit with previous published work in this area, for example the notion of patients as experts, and the stigma attached to having asthma.[28]

In summary, this study has addressed two questions: Do professionals and patients describe asthma in different ways, and what can be inferred from this data about the knowledge base upon which these expressions are constructed? We address each of these in turn.

DO PROFESSIONALS AND PATIENTS DESCRIBE ASTHMA IN DIFFERENT WAYS?

The data show clear areas of congruence or shared understanding between the professionals and the patients: both groups broadly agreed on the treatments for asthma, and agreed that there were difficulties in the use of inhaled steroids. Within the set of data describing the role of steroids, a paradox begins to emerge, elicited particularly by a doctor's use of the phrase "keeps you better for tomorrow". In general, the data suggest that the professionals stressed the prospective benefits from using steroids. Patient participants evaluated the efficacy of the inhaled steroid in the context of their accumulated personal experience of it—ie retrospectively—and judged its value accordingly. We interpret this as evidence of a divergence or "duality" in respect of the two perspectives upon which their respective treatment strategies are based.

A second paradox emerges in the data describing expertise in asthma, and locus of control. A clear theme in the patients' data suggests a developing personal expertise in asthma management, allowing the patient "to advise myself better", or "know my asthma better than anybody". The health care professionals on the other hand, clearly feel a sense of responsibility for managing asthma for patients: they adopt the role of teacher and assume initial responsibility for the disease before deciding, at times, to "put control onto the person". We suggest this might represent a further duality in relation to disease management.

We postulate that these differences in approach to treatment and management imply deeper differences in the ways the two groups think about asthma. That these differences are linked to language is supported by the different metaphors—process versus container noted in their descriptions of the disease. Such a disparity between doctors and patients in the use of metaphor when discussing asthma has recently been highlighted,[11] and reflects an increasing interest in language-based medical research.[29]

WHAT CAN BE INFERRED FROM THIS DATA ABOUT THE KNOWLEDGE BASE UPON WHICH THESE EXPRESSIONS ARE CONSTRUCTED?

This analysis supports the possibility that there is an epistemological difference between doctors and patients in this context. While some might consider this a truism, that the two have different perspectives, we postulate that this may reflect a more profound distinction, namely that each group draws on different types of knowledge to construct the thoughts and words with which they describe asthma. The possibility of such a distinction is recognised in the philosophical literature. We can begin to understand these differences by drawing on Piaget's distinction between figurative and operational knowledge, referred to earlier.[18] The professionals, who in general do not have direct experience of actually having asthma, use their theoretically based knowledge to participate in the dialogue. Piaget would call this type of knowledge operational. The patients' knowledge arises out of direct lived experience, which Piaget classes as figurative. Although these categories are not meant to be mutually exclusive, it does introduces the possibility, arising from the data, that the two groups construe asthma in slightly different ways. Using Toulmin's taxonomy,[20] the professionals draw on universal knowledge, while their patient counterparts use an "existential knowledge base". Again, Byron Good argues that medicine reconstitutes the familiar human body as "the medical body": doctors see the human body in medicine's own way, with medicine's gaze, and use a particular vocabulary to describe it.[30] [31] Within medicine, Good argues, the human body is "newly constituted as a medical body, quite distinct from the bodies with which we interact in everyday life".[30] We argue that in this data set, the words, constructs, and strategies described by the two groups reflect the epistemological dualities postulated by these commentators.

What are the implications of such a view? Firstly, it underlines the relevance of the philosophical literature to everyday clinical practice. Secondly, it demands a "post-modern" view of illness in which the biomedical component is inextricably intertwined with the cultural, societal aspects: no one component is more robust, more real or more relevant. The experience of illness occurs at their intersection."[32] [33] Thirdly, it introduces a potential impediment to implementation: if consultations cannot be seen as literally shared dialogues, but rather as a kind of fluid elusive exchange of extracts from differing knowledge bases, the process of implementation may not be a simple linear process (that is just explaining and handing over information), but may be more complex.

Further research in this area would refine the analytical approach in this study by examining video recordings of live consultations, and interviewing the participants to find out precisely what they were thinking when they made a contribution. Language-based medical research should be encouraged to explore the epistemological basis of patients' and health care professionals' interactions during consultations.

Authors' note

Drs Halpin and Stead had the original idea for the project, assisted in its planning and commented on the article through each of the drafts. Dr Sweeney carried out all the focus groups work and the first level data analysis. Dr Edwards carried out the analysis of the use of metaphor, and commented on the successive drafts of the paper.

Funding

This study arose out of a larger study funded by the NHS National R and D Programme on Asthma Management.

Acknowledgments

We wish to thank Mrs Helene Talbot for her help in identifying the patients and administering the collation of the focus groups, Mrs Annie Hills for her secretarial support, and Drs Sindy Banga and Maggie Cormack for their helpful analysis of a sample of the transcripts.

K G Sweeney, MA, MPhil, MRCGP, is Lecturer, Research and Development Support Unit, School of Postgraduate Medicine and Health Sciences, University of Exeter. Karen Edwards, PhD, is Lecturer, School of English and American Studies, University of Exeter. Dr Jonathan Stead, MPhil, MRCGP, is Consultant in Clinical Effectiveness, North and East Devon Health Authority. Dr David Halpin, DPhil, MRCP, is Senior Lecturer in Respiratory Medicine, School of Postgraduate Medicine and Health Sciences, University of Exeter.

References

1 Hilton S, Anderson HR, Sibbald B, Freeling P. Controlled evaluation of the effects of patient centred education on asthma morbidity in general practice. *Lancet* 1986;i:26-9.
2 Turner-Warwick M. Nocturnal asthma: a study in general practice. *Journal of the Royal College of General Practitioners* 1989;39:239-43.
3 Horn CR, Cochraine GM. An audit of morbidity associated with chronic asthma in general practice. *Respiratory Medicine* 1989;83:71-5.
4 Dudbridge SB, Stead J, Ward S, Amooie M, Halpin DMG. The Devon primary care asthma initiative: effects on morbidity. *American Journal of Respiratory Critical Care Medicine* 1996;153: A868.
5 Charlton IH, Charlton G, Broomfield J, Mullee MA. The effect of nurse run asthma clinic on workload and patient morbidity in general practice. *British Journal of General Practice* 1991;41: 227-31.
6 Jones KP, Bain DJG, Middleton M, Mullee MA. Correlates of asthma morbidity in primary care. *British Medical Journal* 1992;304:361-4.
7 Jones KP, Charlton IH, Middleton M, Preece WJ, Hill AP. Targeting asthma care in general practice using a morbidity index. *British Medical Journal* 1992;304:1353-6.
8 O'Connor GT, Weiss ST. Clinical and symptom measures. *American Journal of Respiratory Critical Care Medicine* 1994;149: S21-8.
9 Morris NV, Abrahamson MJ, Strusser RP. Adequacy of control of asthma in general practice. Is maximum peak expiratory flow rate a valid index of asthma severity? *Medical Journal of Australia* 1994;160:68-71.
10 Apter AJ, Zu Wallack RL, Clive J. Common measures of asthma severity lack association for describing its clinical course. *Journal of Allergy and Immunology* 1994;94:732-7.
11 Atherton A, Tyrrell Z, White PT. *Perception and reported use of inhaled steroids in primary care* [report to Department of Health]. London: King's College, 1998.
12 Adams S, Pill R, Jones A. Medication chronic illness and identity: the perspective of people with asthma. *Social Science and Medicine* 1997;45:189-202.
13 Ostergaard MS. Childhood asthma: parents' perspective, a qualitative interview study *Family Practice* 1998;15:153-7.
14 Johnson M, Lackoff G. *Metaphors we live by.* Chicago University of Chicago Press, 1980.
15 Mabeck CE, Oleson F. Metaphorically transmitted diseases. How do patients embody medical explanations? *Family Practice* 1997;14:271-8.
16 Leary D, ed. *Metaphors in the history of psychology.* Cambridge University of Cambridge Press, 1994.
17 Beate D, Skorpen J, Malterud K. What did the doctor say–what did the patient do: operational knowledge in clinical communication. *Family Practice* 1997;4:376-81.
18 Piaget J. *The language and thought of the child.* London, Kegan Paul, Trench Trubener, 1932.
19 Silverman H J, ed. *Piaget, philosophy and the human sciences.* Evanston, Illinois: Northwestern University Press, 1980.
20 Toulmin S. Knowledge and art in the practice of medicine: clinical judgment and historical reconstruction. In: Delkeshamp-Hayes C, Gardell Cutter MAG, eds. *Science, technology and the art of medicine. European-American Dialogues.* Dordrecht: Kluwer, 1993.
21 Polanyi M. *Personal knowledge.* London: Routledge and Kegan Paul, 1973.
22 Morgan DL. *Focus groups in qualitative research.* London: Sage Publications, 1988.
23 Denzin NK, Lincoln YS, eds. *Handbook of qualitative research.* Thousand Oaks, California: Sage, 1994.
24 Holloway I. *Basic concepts in qualitative research.* London: Blackwell Press, 1997.
25 Miles MP, Hubermann AM. *Qualitative analysis: an expanded source book.* London: Sage Publications, 1994.
26 Sweeney KG. *The use of focus groups to assess consumers' views on miscarriage and minor surgery* [MPhil thesis]. Exeter: University of Exeter,1996.
27 Adams S, Pill R, Jones A. Medication, chronic illness and identity: the perspective of people with asthma. *Social Science and Medicine* 1997;45:189-210.
28 Goffman E. *Stigma: notes on the management of spoiled identity.* Harmondsworth: Penguin, 1968.
29 Skelton JR, Hobbs FDR. Concordancing: use of language based research in medical communication. *Lancet* 1999;353: 108-11.
30 Good B. *Medicine, rationality and experience.* Cambridge: Cambridge University Press, 1994.
31 Evans M The "medical body" as philosophy's arena. *Theoretical Medicine and Bioethics* 2001(in press).
32 Morris D. *Illness and Culture in the Postmodern Age.* California, University of California Press, 1998..
33 Muir Gray JA. Postmodern medicine. *Lancet* 1999;354:1550-13.

References and further reading

References

Adorno T, Albert H, Dahrendors R, Habermas J, Piloth B, Popper K (1976) *The Positivist Dispute in German Sociology*. Heinemann, London.

American Board of Internal Medicine (1985) *Subcommittee of the Evaluation of Humanistic Qualities in the Internist. A guide to awareness and evaluation*. American Board of Internal Medicine, Washington, DC.

Anon. (1995) Evidence-based medicine, in its place. *Lancet.* **346**: 785.

Armenian HK, Lilienfield DE (1994) Applications of the case–control method: overview and historical perspective. *Epidemiol Rev.* **16**: 1–5.

Armstrong D, Reyburn H, Jones R (1996) A study of general practitioners' reasons for changing their prescribing behaviour. *BMJ.* **312**: 494–5.

Aron R (1970) *Main Currents in Sociological Thought*. Penguin, Harmondsworth.

Ashby R (1952) *Design for a Brain*. John Wiley & Sons, New York.

Bacon F (1858) *The Works of Francis Bacon, Baron of Verulam, Viscount St Alban, and Lord High Chancellor of England*. Longman & Co., London.

Bailey C (1947) *Titus Lucretius Carus: de natura rerum*. Oxford University Press, Oxford.

Balint M (1957) *The Doctor, his Patient, and the Illness*. International Universities Press, New York.

Battram A (1998) *Navigating Complexity*. The Industrial Society, London.

Baxt WG (1994) Complexity chaos and human physiology: the justification for non-linear neural computational analysis. *Cancer Lett.* **77**: 85–93.

Becker MH (1974) The health belief model and sick role of behaviour. *Health Educ Monogr.* **2**: 409–19.

Berkeley G (1967) *The Principles of Human Knowledge*. Fontana, London.

Bloor M (1976) Bishop Berkeley and the adeno-tonsillectomy enigma: an exploration in the social construction on medical disposals. *Sociology.* **10**: 43–51.

Boston Area Anticoagulation Trial for Atrial Fibrillation Investigators (1990) The effects of low-dose warfarin on the risk of stroke in patients with non-rheumatic atrial fibrillation. *NEJM.* **323**: 1505–11.

Bradley F, Field I (1995) Evidence-based medicine (letter). *Lancet.* **346**: 838–9.

Briggs J, Peat FD (1989) *Turbulent Mirror*. Harper and Row, New York.

British Medical Association (2003) *New GMS Contract. Investing in general practice*. NHS Confederation, London.

Brock W (1985) *From Prototype to Proton: William Prout and the nature of matter, 1785–1985*. Hilger, Bristol.

Brock WH (1993) The biochemical tradition. In: Bynum WF, Porter R (eds) *Companion Encyclopaedia of the History of Medicine*. Routledge, London.

Brook R, Kosecoff JB, Park RE *et al.* (1988) Diagnosis and treatment of coronary disease: a comparison of doctors' attitudes in the UK and USA. *Lancet.* **1**: 750–3.

Brown JR (2001) *Who Rules in Science?* Harvard University Press, Cambridge, MA.

Bunker J (1995) Medicine matters after all. *J R Coll Physicians.* **29**: 105–12.

Burke P (1981) *Montaigne*. Oxford University Press, Oxford.

Burnand B, Kernan WN, Feinstein AR (1990) Indexes and boundaries for 'quantitative significance' in statistical decisions. *J Clin Epidemiol.* **43**: 1273–84.

Bynum WF, Porter R (eds) (1993) *Companion Encyclopaedia to the History of Medicine.* Routledge, London.

Byron A, Boyd C (1991) *Rudolf Virchow: the scientist as citizen.* Garland, New York.

Cannon WB (1939) *The Wisdom of the Body.* Norton, New York.

Capra F (1983) *The Turning Point: science, society and the rising culture.* Flamingo, New York.

Capra F (1996) *The Web of Life.* Doubleday, New York.

Cartwright A, Anderson R (1981) *General Practice Revisited: a second study of patients and their doctors.* Tavistock, London.

Casti JL (1995) *Complexification.* Harper Perennial, New York.

Centre for Disease Control (2000) *Centre for Disease Control Daily News* (accessed 22 September 2000); www.ama-assn.org/special/hiv/newsline/cdd/091800g3.html.

Chalmers AF (1982) *What is This Thing Called Science?* Open University Press, Buckingham.

Charlton BG (1995a) Megatrials are subordinate to medical science (letter). *BMJ.* **311:** 257.

Charlton R (1995b) Balancing science and art in primary care research: past and present. *Br J Gen Pract.* **45:** 639–40.

Cilliers P (1998) *Complexity and Postmodernism.* Routledge, London.

Cochrane AL (1971) *Effectiveness and Efficiency: random reflections on health services.* Nuffield Provincial Hospital Trust (Rock Carling Fellowship), London.

Cohen J, Stewart I (1994) *The Collapse of Chaos.* Penguin, Harmondsworth.

Collingwood RG (1946) *The Idea of History.* Clarendon Press, Oxford.

Collins R, Peto R, Gray R *et al.* (1996) In: Weatherall DJ, Ledingham JGG, Warrell DA (eds) *The Oxford Textbook of Medicine.* Oxford University Press, Oxford.

Comte A (1875) (trans. Martineau H) (1974) *The Positive Philosophy.* Ams Press, New York.

Comte A (1993) In: Microsoft *Encarta Encyclopaedia.* Funk and Wagnalls, Seattle.

Connolly SJ, Laupacis A, Gent M *et al.* (1991) Canadian Atrial Fibrillation Anticoagulation (CAFA) Study. *J Am Cardiol.* **18:** 349–55.

Creswell JW (1988) *Qualitative Enquiry and Research Design.* Sage Publications, London.

Cromarty I (1996) What do patients think about during their consultations? A qualitative study. *Br J Gen Pract.* **46:** 525–8.

Crosby A (1997) *The Measure of Reality: quantification in Western society 1250–1600.* Cambridge University Press, New York.

Cunningham A (1989) Thomas Sydenham: epidemics, experiments and the good old cause. In: French R, Wear A (eds) *The Medical Revolution in the Seventeenth Century.* Cambridge University Press, Cambridge.

Darlington S (2000) *Brazil Becomes Model in AIDS Fight* (accessed 7 November 2000); www.aegis.org/news/re/2000/re001107.html.

Davidoff F, Haynes B, Sackett D *et al.* (1995) Evidence-based medicine (editorial). *BMJ.* **310:** 1085–6.

Dawes MG (1996) On the need for evidence-based general and family practice. *Evidence-Based Med.* **1:** 68–9.

Delblanco A (2001) Night vision. Review of *The Moral Obligation to be Intelligent: selected essays* by L Trilling. *New York Rev Books.* **48.**

Denzin NK, Lincoln YS (1994) *A Handbook of Qualitative Research.* Sage Publications, Thousand Oaks, CA.

Department of Health (1962) *A Hospital Plan for England and Wales.* HMSO, London.

Department of Health (1972) *Report of the Working Party on Medical Administrators. The Grey Book.* HMSO, London.

Department of Health and Social Security (1983) *NHS Management Enquiry: Griffiths Report.* Department of Health and Social Security, London.

Descartes R (trans. Veitch A) (1912) *A Discourse on Method: meditations and principles.* Dent & Sons Ltd, London.

Devor E J (1993) Genetic disease. In: Kiple K (ed.) *The Cambridge History of Human Disease.* Cambridge University Press, Cambridge.

Dilman I (1973) *Induction and Deduction: a study in Wittgenstein.* Basil Blackwell, Oxford.

Dixon M, Sweeney KG (2000) *The Human Effect in Medicine: theory, research and practice.* Radcliffe Medical Press, Oxford.

Doll R, Hill AB (1950) Smoking and carcinoma of the lung: preliminary report. *BMJ.* **ii:** 1225–36.

Dubos R (1960) *The Mirage of Health.* George Allen & Unwin, London.

Dunn J, Urmson JO, Ayer AJ (1992) *The British Empiricists. Locke, Berkeley, Hume.* Oxford University Press, Oxford.

Durie R, Wyatt K, Fox M, Sweeney K (2004) *Receptive Context in the Pursuing Perfection Programme. Report for the Modernisation Agency of the Department of Health.* Health Complexity Group, Exeter.

Ellis J, Mulligan I, Rowe J *et al.* (1995) In-patient general medicine is evidence based. *Lancet.* **346:** 407–10.

Elstein AS, Kagan N, Hulman D *et al.* (1972) Methods and theory in the study of medical inquiry. *J Med Educ.* **47:** 85–92.

Engel GL (1977) The need for a new medical model: a challenge for biomedicine. *Science.* **196:** 129–36.

European Atrial Fibrillation Study Group (1993) Secondary prevention in non-rheumatic atrial fibrillation after transient ischaemic attack or minor stroke. *Lancet.* **342:** 1255–62.

Evans M, Sweeney KG (1998) *The Human Side of Medicine.* Occasional Paper No. 72. Royal College of General Practitioners, London.

Evidence-Based Medicine Working Group (1992) Evidence-based medicine: a new approach to teaching the practice of medicine. *JAMA.* **268:** 2420–5.

Ezekowitz MD, Bridgers SL, James KE *et al.* for the Veterans Affairs Stroke Prevention in Non-Rheumatic Atrial Fibrillation Investigators (1992) Warfarin in the prevention of stroke associated with non-rheumatic atrial fibrillation. *NEJM.* **327:** 1406–12.

Fahey T, Schroder K (2004) Recent advances in primary care: cardiology. *Br J Gen Pract.* **54:** 696–703.

Feinstein AR (1992) Insidious comparisons and unmet clinical challenges. *Am J Med.* **92:** 117–20.

Feinstein AR (2002) Will clinicians' challenges be solved by another theoretical model? Commentary on Sweeney and Kernick (2002) Clinical evaluation: constructing a new model for post-normal medicine. *J Clin Evaluation.* **8:** 139–41.

Fishbein M, Azjen I (1975) *Belief, Attitude, Intention and Behavior.* John Wiley & Sons, New York.

Fletcher R (1971) *The Making of Sociology: a study of sociological theory. Volume 1.* Michael Joseph, London.

Foucault M (1963) *The Birth of the Clinic.* Tavistock, London.

Fowler PBS (1995) Evidence-based medicine (letter). *Lancet.* **346:** 838.

Fraser S, Greenhalgh T (2001) Coping with complexity: educating for capability. *BMJ.* **323:** 799–802.

Fraser SW, Conner M, Yarrow D (eds) (2003) *Thriving in Unpredictable Times: a reader on agility in health care.* Kingsham Press, Chichester.

Freeman A, Sweeney K (2001) Why general practitioners do not implement evidence: a qualitative study. *BMJ.* **323:** 1100–14.

Freund J (1968) *The Sociology of Max Weber.* Allen Lane, London.

Fukuyama F (1993) *The End of History and the Last Man.* Penguin, Harmondsworth.

Garfinkel A, Spano ML, Ditto WL, Weiss JN (1992) Controlling cardiac chaos. *Science.* **257:** 1230–5.

Garratini S, Garratini L (1993) Pharmaceutical prescribing in four European countries. *Lancet.* **342:** 1191–2.

Geyer R (2001) *Beyond the Third Way: the science of complexity and the politics of choice.* Paper presented to the Joint Session of the ECPR, Grenoble, April 2001.

Giddens A (1974) *Positivism and Sociology*. Heinemann Educational, London.

Gill P, Dowell AC, Neal RD *et al.* (1996) Evidence-based general practice: a retrospective study of interventions in one training practice. *BMJ.* **312:** 819–21.

Gillies J (2005) *Getting it Right in the Consultation. Hippocrates' problem, Aristotle's answer.* Occasional Paper No. 86. Royal College of General Practitioners, London.

Gillon R, Wesley S (1998) Medicalisation of distress. *R Soc Arts J.* **4:** 80–6.

Gleick J (1998) *Chaos*. Vintage, London.

Gloubermann S, Zimmerman B (2002) *Complicated and Complex Systems: what would successful reform of Medicare look like?* Discussion Paper No. 8. Commission on the Future of Health Care in Canada, Montreal.

Goldberger AL, West BJ (1987) Applications of non-linear dynamics to clinical cardiology. *Ann N Y Acad Sci.* **504:** 195–213.

Grbich C (1999) *Qualitative Research in Health*. Sage Publications, Thousand Oaks, CA.

Greaves D (1996) *Mystery in Western Medicine*. Ashgate Publishing Ltd, Aldershot.

Greenhalgh T (1996) Is my practice evidence-based? *BMJ.* **313:** 957–8.

Greenhalgh T (2002) Intuition and evidence: uneasy bedfellows? *Br J Gen Pract.* **52:** 395–400.

Gribbin J (2004) *Deep Simplicity*. Allen Lane, London.

Griffiths F (2002) Complexity and primary healthcare research. In: Sweeney K, Griffiths F (eds) *Complexity and Healthcare: an introduction*. Radcliffe Medical Press, Oxford.

Grimshaw JM, Russell IT (1993) Effect of clinical guidelines on medical practice: a systematic review of rigorous evaluations. *Lancet.* **342:** 1317–22.

Guilbert JJ (1987) Educational objectives. In: *Educational Handbook for Health Care Personnel*. World Health Organization, Geneva.

Guyatt GH, Rennie D (1993) Users' guides to the medical literature. *JAMA.* **270:** 2096–7.

Guyatt GH, Sackett DL, Cook DJ (1994) Users' guides to the medical literature. II. How to use an article about therapy or prevention. *JAMA.* **271:** 59–63.

Haines A, Jones R (1994) Implementing findings in research. *BMJ.* **308:** 1488–92.

Hammer M (1995) *The Re-Engineering Revolution*. Harper Business, New York.

Haraway DJ (1976) *Crystals, Fabrics and Fields: metaphors of organicism in twentieth-century developmental biology*. Yale University Press, New Haven, CT.

Harrison S (1988) *Managing the NHS: shifting the frontier?* Chapman and Hall, London.

Harrison T (1947) The future of sociology. *Pilot Papers.* **2:** 10–21.

Hassey A (2002) Complexity and the clinical encounter. In: Sweeney K, Griffiths F (eds) (2002) *Complexity and Healthcare: an introduction*. Radcliffe Medical Press, Oxford.

Hawthorn G (1976) *Enlightenment and Despair: a history of sociology*. Cambridge University Press, Cambridge.

Health Complexity Group (2004) *Creating an Enabling Context for Change: linking research to practical examples of quality improvement*. Workshop presented at the European Quality Forum, Copenhagen, June 2004.

Heath I (1995) *The Mystery of General Practice*. Nuffield Provincial Hospitals Trust, London.

Heisenberg W (1971) *Physics and Beyond*. Harper and Row, New York.

Holland JH (1998) *From Chaos to Order*. Oxford University Press, Oxford.

Holloway I (1997) *Basic Concepts for Qualitative Research*. Blackwell Science, Oxford.

Holt T (2002a) A tight model for diabetes control. *Diabet Med.* **19:** 274–8.

Holt T (2002b) Clinical knowledge, chaos and complexity. In: Sweeney K, Griffiths F (eds) *Complexity and Healthcare: an introduction*. Radcliffe Medical Press, Oxford.

Honderich T (ed.) (1995) *The Oxford Companion to Philosophy*. Oxford University Press, Oxford.

Howie JGR (1972) Diagnosis: the Achilles' heel? *J R Coll Gen Pract.* **22:** 310–15.

Howie JGR, Bigg AR (1980) Family trends in psychotropic and antibiotic prescribing in general practice. *BMJ.* **280:** 836–8.

Hughes H (1959) *Consciousness and Society: the real orientation of European social thought 1890–1930*. MacGibbon and Kee, London.

Hume D. *Enquiries Concerning Human Understanding and Concerning the Principles of Morals* (3e) (1975). Oxford University Press, Oxford.

Hume D (1739) *A Treatise on Human Nature* (2e) (1978). Clarendon Press, Oxford.

Iggo N (1995) Evidence-based medicine (letter). *Lancet.* **346:** 839.

Illich I (1975) *Medical Nemesis: the expropriation of health.* Calder and Boyars, London.

Johnson M (1995) Health-related behaviour change. In: *Preventing Coronary Heart Disease in Primary Care.* King's Fund, London.

Kaplan SH, Greenfield S, Ware JE (1989) Assessing the effects of physician–patient interactions on the outcomes of chronic disease. *Med Care.* **27 (suppl. 3):** S110–27.

Kauffman S (1993) *The Origins of Order.* Oxford University Press, New York.

Kember T, MacPherson G (1994) *The NHS: a kaleidoscope of care – conflict of service and business values.* Nuffield Hospitals Provincial Trust, London.

Kernick D (2002) Complexity and healthcare organisation. In: Sweeney K, Griffiths F (eds) *Complexity and Healthcare: an introduction.* Radcliffe Medical Press, Oxford.

Kernick D, Sweeney K (2001) Post normal medicine (editorial). *Fam Pract.* **18:** 356–8.

King LS (1982) *Medical Thinking: a historical preface.* Princeton University Press, Princeton, NJ.

Kirkpatrick B (ed.) (1994) *Concise English Dictionary.* Cassell, London.

Klein R (1989) *The Politics of the NHS* (2e). Longman, London.

Kleinman A (1988) *The Illness Narrative.* Basic Books, New York.

Koch R (1891) Ueber Bakteriologische Forschung. In: *Verhandlungen des X Internationalen Medicinischen Congresses, Berlin, 4–9 August 1890.* Hirschwald, Berlin.

Kuhn TS (1970) *The Structure of Scientific Revolutions.* University of Chicago Press, Chicago.

Landau RL, Gustaffson JM (1984) Death is not the enemy. *JAMA.* **252:** 2458.

Laupacis A (1993) Anticoagulants for atrial fibrillation (editorial). *Lancet.* **343:** 1251.

Laupacis A, Wells G, Richardson SW, Tugwell P (1994) Users' guides to the medical literature. V. How to use an article about prognosis. *JAMA.* **272:** 234–7.

Le Fanu J (1999) *The Rise and Fall of Modern Medicine.* Abacus, London.

Lilford RJ, Braunholtz D (1996) The statistical basis of public policy: a paradigm shift is overdue. *BMJ.* **313:** 603–7.

Lilienfield AM, Lilienfield DE (1979) A century of case-controlled studies: progress? *J Chron Dis.* **32:** 5–13.

Lilienfield DE, Stolley PD (1994) *Foundations of Epidemiology* (3e). Oxford University Press, New York.

Liska-Hackzell JJ (1999) Predictions of blood glucose levels in diabetic patients using a hybrid AI technique. *Comput Biomed Res.* **32:** 132–44.

Lorenz EN (1963) Deterministic non-periodic flow. *J Atmosph Sci.* **20:** 130–41.

Lowe GDO (1993) Antithrombotic treatment and atrial fibrillation (editorial). *BMJ.* **305:** 1445–6.

McColl A, Smith H, White P, Field J (1998) General practitioners' perceptions of the route to evidence-based medicine: a questionnaire survey. *BMJ.* **316:** 361–5.

McWhinney IR (1983) Changing models: the impact of Kuhn's theory on medical practice. *Fam Pract.* **1:** 3–8.

Malinowski B (1922) *Argonauts of the Western Pacific.* Routledge, London.

Marinker M (1970) Balint seminars and vocational training in general practice. *J R Coll Gen Pract.* **19:** 79.

Marinker M (1981) Clinical method. In: Cormack J, Marinker M, Morrell D (eds) *Teaching Clinical Method.* Kluwer Medical, London.

Marinker M (1994) *The End of General Practice (Bayliss Lecture).* Royal College of Physicians, London.

Mass Observation (1938) *First Year's Work.* Lindsay Drummond, London.

Mass Observation (1949) *Meet Yourself at the Doctor's.* Naldrett Press, London.

Mears R, Sweeney K (2000) A preliminary study of the decision-making process within general practice. *Fam Pract.* **17:** 428–9.

Midgley M (1992) *Science as Salvation: a modern myth and its meaning.* Routledge, London.

Mill J (1974) *A System of Logic: being a connected view of the principles of evidence and methods of scientific investigation.* University of Toronto Press, Toronto.

Mitelton-Kelly E (2003) Ten principles of complexity and enabling infrastructures. In: Mitelton-Kelly E (ed.) *Complex Systems and Evolutionary Perspectives of Organisations: applications of complexity theory to organisations.* Elsevier, London.

Mitelton-Kelly E (2004) *The Principles of Complex Evolving Systems.* Presentation to the Fourth Exeter Complexity Conference, September 2004, Exeter.

Mitelton-Kelly E, Papefthimiou B (2000) *The Bank Case Study. International Workshop on Feedback and Evolution in Software and Business Processes (FEAST),* July 2000, London.

Morris DB (1998) *Illness and Culture in a Postmodern Age.* University of California Press, Berkeley, CA.

Murphy E, Dingwall R, Greatbatch D, Parker S, Watson P (1998) *Qualitative Research Methods in Health Technology Assessment: a review of the literature.* Health Technology Assessment, NHS R&D HTA Programme, London.

NHS Management Executive (1992) *First Steps Towards the New NHS.* Department of Health, London.

Neighbour R (1987) *The Inner Consultation.* MTP Press, Lancaster.

Oxman AD, Sackett DL, Guyatt GH (1993) Users' guides to the medical literature. I. How to get started. *JAMA.* **270:** 2093–5.

Pederson S (2005) Anti-condescensionism. *London Rev Books.* 1 **September:** 7–8.

Peppiatt R (1992) Eliciting patients' views of the cause of their problems: a practical strategy for GPs. *Fam Pract.* **9:** 295–8.

Petersen P, Boysen G, Godtfredsen J, Andersen ED, Andersen B (1989) Placebo-controlled randomised trial of warfarin and aspirin for prevention of thromboembolic complications in chronic atrial fibrillation: the Copenhagen AFASAK study. *Lancet.* **1:** 175–9.

Phillips ED (1973) *Greek Medicine.* Thames and Hudson, London.

Piaget J (1932) *The Language and Thought of the Child.* Kegan Paul, London.

Pinchot G, Pinchot E (1996) *The Intelligent Organisation: engaging the talent and initiative of everyone in the workplace.* Berrett-Koehler, San Francisco, CA.

Plato (trans.) (1979) *The Sophist.* Garland, New York.

Plsek P (2000) *Crossing the Quality Chasm: a new health system for the twenty-first century.* National Academy Press, Washington, DC.

Plsek P (2002) Foreword. In: Sweeney K, Griffiths F (eds) *Complexity and Healthcare: an introduction.* Radcliffe Medical Press, Oxford.

Plsek P, Wilson T (2001) Complexity, leadership and management in healthcare organisations. *BMJ.* **323:** 746–9.

Poincare H (1952) *Science and Hypothesis.* Dover, New York.

Poincare H (1958) *Science and Value.* Dover, New York.

Polanyi M (1958) *Personal Knowledge: towards a post critical philosophy.* University of Chicago Press, Chicago.

Popper KR (1963) *The Open Society and its Enemies.* Princeton University Press, Princeton, NJ.

Porter R (1987) *A Social History of Madness.* Weidenfeld and Nicholson, London.

Porter R (1997) *The Greatest Benefit to Mankind.* Fontana, London.

Pradilla R (1992) *Qualitative and quantitative models of social situations: the case for triangulation of paradigms.* International Symposium on Qualitative Research Process and Computing, Bremen, Germany.

Prein G (1992) *Traps of triangulation: what can be done by combining qualitative and quantitative methods?* International Symposium on Qualitative Research Process and Computing, Bremen, Germany.

Prigogine I (1998) *The End of Certainty: time chaos and the new laws of nature.* The Free Press, New York.

Puustinen M (2000) What is medicine? In search for (*sic*) a theory of practice. In: Louhala P, Stenman S (eds) *Philosophy Meets Medicine*. Helsinki University Press, Helsinki.

Rassam SM (1993) Anticoagulation in patients with atrial fibrillation (letter). *BMJ*. **307:** 1492.

Reiser SJ (1991) *Medicine and the Reign of Technology*. Cambridge University Press, Cambridge.

Robinson R, LeGrand J (1994) *Evaluating the NHS Reforms*. King's Fund, London.

Rogers EM (1983) *Diffusion of Innovations*. The Free Press, New York.

Rosenberg W, Donald A (1995) Evidence-based medicine: an approach to clinical problem solving. *BMJ*. **310:** 1122–6.

Ross D (trans.) (1988, revised) *Aristotle: the Nicomachean ethics*. Oxford University Press, Oxford.

Rossler OE, Rossler R (1994) Chaos in physiology. *Integr Physiol Behav Sci* **29:** 328–33.

Rossman GWB (1985) Numbers and words: combining qualitative and quantitative methods in a single large-scale evaluation study. *Evaluation Rev.* **9:** 627–43.

Royal College of General Practitioners (1972) *The Future General Practitioner. Learning and teaching*. Royal College of General Practitioners, London.

Rudebeck CE (1992) Humanism in medicine: benevolence or realism? *Scand J Prim Health Care.* **10:** 161–2.

Ruse M (1995) In: Honderich T (ed.) (1995) *The Oxford Companion to Philosophy*. Oxford University Press, Oxford.

Russell B (1961) *The History of Western Philosophy*. Unwin Paperbacks, London.

Sackett DL, Cook RJ (1994) Understanding clinical trials (editorial). *BMJ*. **309:** 755–6

Sackett DL, Rosenberg WM (1995) The need for evidence-based medicine. *J R Soc Med.* **88:** 620–4.

Sackett DL, Haines RB, Tugwell P (1985) *Clinical Epidemiology: a Basic Science for Clinical Medicine*. Little & Brown, Boston, MA.

Sackett DL, Rosenberg WM, Gray JA, Haynes RB, Richardson WS (1996) Evidence-based medicine: what it is and what it isn't. *BMJ*. **312:** 71–2.

Schaffer WM (1985) Can non-linear dynamics elucidate mechanisms in ecology and epidemiology? *IMA J Math Appl Med Biol.* **2:** 221–52.

Schneider L (1967) *The Scottish Moralists on Human Nature and Society*. University of Chicago Press, Chicago.

Scruton R (1982) *Kant*. Oxford University Press, Oxford.

Second International Study of Infarct Survival Collaborative Group (1988) Randomised trial of intravenous streptokinase, oral aspirin, both or neither among 17 187 cases of suspected acute myocardial infarction. *Lancet.* **ii:** 349–60.

Silagy C, Jewell D (1994) Review of 39 years of randomised controlled trials in the *British Journal of General Practice*. *Br J Gen Pract.* **44:** 359–63.

Singer C, Underwood EA (1962) *A Short History of Medicine* (2e). Clarendon Press, Oxford.

Skrabanek P, McCormick J (1989) *Follies and Fallacies in Medicine*. Tarragon Press, Chippenham.

Smeeth L, Haines A, Ebrahim S (1999) Numbers needed to treat derived from meta-analyses – sometimes informative, usually misleading. *BMJ*. **318:** 1548–51.

Smith A (1776) *An Enquiry into the Nature and Causes of the Wealth of Nations* (1976). University of Chicago Press, Chicago.

Smith A (1993) In: Microsoft *Encarta Encyclopaedia*. Funk and Wengells, Seattle.

Smith BH (1995) Quality cannot always be quantified (letter). *BMJ*. **311:** 258.

Smith J, Heshusius L (1986) Closing down the conversation: the end of the quantitative–qualitative debate among educational enquirers. *Educ Researcher.* **15:** 4–12.

Snowden D (2002) *Story Telling, Narrative Analysis and Transformational Change in Multi-National Corporations*. Presentation at the Second Exeter Complexity Conference, Exeter, September 2002.

Southgate L, Jolly B (1994) Determining the content of re-certification procedures. In: Newble D, Wakeford R, Jolly B (eds) *The Certification and Re-Certification of Doctors.* Cambridge University Press, Cambridge.

Stacey R (2000) *Strategic Management and Organisational Dynamics: the challenge of complexity.* Financial Times, London.

Stacey R (2001) *Complex Responsive Processes in Organisations.* Routledge, London.

Stalking G (1995) *After Taylor: British socio-anthropology, 1888–1951.* University of Wisconsin Press, Madison, WI.

Starfield B (2001) New paradigms for quality in primary care. *Br J Gen Pract.* **51**: 303–9.

Stephenson RC (2004) Using a complexity model of human behaviour to help inter-professional clinical reasoning. *Int J Ther Rehabil.* **11**: 168–75.

Stewart I (1989) *Does God Play Dice?* Blackwell, Cambridge, MA.

Stroke Prevention in Atrial Fibrillation Investigators (1991) Stroke prevention in atrial fibrillation study: final results. *Circulation.* **84**: 527–39.

Sweeney BJ (1992) *Is there an expertise in human relationship?* (MPhil thesis). University of Glasgow, Glasgow.

Sweeney KG (1996) Evidence and uncertainty. In: Marinker M (ed.) *Sense and Sensibility in Healthcare.* BMJ Publishing, London.

Sweeney K (2003a) Progressing clinical governance through complexity: from managing to co-creating. In: Kernick D (ed.) *Complexity and Healthcare Organisations.* Radcliffe Medical Press, Oxford.

Sweeney K (2003b) *Final Report to the Nuffield Trust for the Health Complexity Group.* Nuffield Trust, London. Unpublished.

Sweeney KG, Griffiths FE (eds) (2002) *Complexity and Healthcare: an introduction.* Radcliffe Medical Press, Oxford.

Sweeney KG, Kernick D (2002) Clinical evaluation: a new model for post normal medicine. *J Eval Clin Pract.* **8**: 131–8.

Sweeney K, Mannion R (2002) Complexity and clinical governance: using the insights to develop the strategy. *Br J Gen Pract.* **52** (Suppl.) S4–9.

Sweeney KG, Pereira Gray DJ, Steele RJ, Evans PH (1995) The use of warfarin in non-rheumatic atrial fibrillation: a commentary from general practice. *Br J Gen Pract.* **45**: 153–8.

Sweeney KG, MacAuley D, Pereira Gray DJ (1998) Personal significance: the third dimension. *Lancet.* **351**: 134–6.

Taylor FW (1911) *Principles of Scientific Management.* Harper & Brothers, New York.

Ten Have HAM (1990) Knowledge and practice in European medicine. The case of infectious diseases. In: Ten Have HAM, Kimsa GK, Spicker SF (eds) *The Growth of Medical Knowledge.* Academic Publishers, Dordrecht.

Tennison B (2002) Complexity and epidemiology in public health. In: Sweeney K, Griffiths (eds) *Complexity and Healthcare: an introduction.* Radcliffe Medical Press, Oxford.

Times (2002) Leading article. *The Times.* 27 June: 1.

Toon P (1994) *What is Good General Practice?* Occasional Paper No. 65. Royal College of General Practitioners, London.

Tuck R (1993) *Philosophy and Government 1572–1651.* Cambridge University Press, Cambridge.

Urry J (1993) *Before Social Anthropology: essays on the history of British anthropology.* Harwood Academic.

Van der Vleuten CP, Newble DI (1995) How can we test clinical reasoning? *Lancet.* **345**: 1032–4.

Virchow R (1895) (trans. Rather LJ) (1958) One hundred years of general pathology. In: *Diseases, Life and Man.* Stanford University Press, Stanford, CA.

Volberda HW, Lewin AY (2003) Co-evolutionary dynamics within and between firms: from evolution to co-evolution. *J Manag Stud.* **40**: 2111–36.

von Bertalanffy L (1968) *General Systems Theory.* Braziller, New York.

von Foerster H, Zoff GW (eds) (1962) *Principles of Self-Organisation.* Pergamon, New York.

Weber M (1963) *'Objectivity' in Social Science and Social Policy.* Random House, New York.

Wheatley M (2000) *Leadership and the New Science.* Berrett Koehler, San Francisco, CA.

Whitehead AN (1929) *Process and Reality.* Macmillan, New York.

Willett C (1999) Knowledge sharing shifts the power paradigm. In: Maybury M, Morey D, Thuraisingham B (eds) *Knowledge Management: classic and contemporary works.* Massachusetts Institute of Technology Press, Cambridge, MA.

Williamson JW, Goldschmidt PG, Jilson IA (1979) *Information Demonstration Project: final report.* Policy Research, Baltimore, MD.

World Bank (1997) *Confronting AIDS: public priorities in a global epidemic;* www.worldbank. org/aids-econ/confrontfull/summary.html.

World Health Organization (2002) *Archives: the World Health Report 2000.* World Health Organization, Geneva.

Wright P, Treacher A (eds) (1982) *The Problem of Medical Knowledge.* Edinburgh University Press, Edinburgh.

Wulff HR (1990) Function and value of medical knowledge in modern diseases. In: Ten Have HAM, Kimsa GK, Spicker SF (eds) *The Growth of Medical Knowledge.* Academic Publishers, Dordrecht.

Yarrow D, Fraser S, Tennison B (2003) Planning and scheduling: maintaining flow in adaptive systems. In: Fraser SW, Conner M, Yarrow D (eds) *Thriving in Unpredictable Times: a reader on agility in health care.* Kingsham Press, Chichester.

Zimmerman B, Plsek P (1998) *Edgeware: insights from complexity science for healthcare leaders.* VHA, Irving.

Zukav G (1979) *The Dancing Wu Li Masters.* Bantam, New York.

Further reading

Abramsom JS, Mizrahi T (1996) When social workers and physicians collaborate: positive and negative interdisciplinary experiences. *Soc Work.* **41**: 270–81.

Adams S, Pill R, Jones A (1997) Medication, chronic illness and identity: the perspective of people with asthma. *Soc Sci Med.* **145**: 189–201.

Anon. (1992) Systematical overview of controlled trials (meta-analysis) helps us to clarify treatment effects. *Drug Ther Bull.* **30**.

Apter AJ, Wallack RL, Clive J (1994) Common measures of asthma severity lack association for describing its clinical course. *J Allergy Immunol.* **94**: 732–7.

Atherton A, Tyrrell A, White PT (1998) *Perception and Reported Use of Inhaled Steroids in Primary Care. Report to Department of Health.* King's College, London.

Barry CA, Bradley CP, Britten N, Stevenson FA, Barber N (2000) Patients' unvoiced agendas in general practice consultations: qualitative study. *BMJ.* **320**: 1246–50.

Barton S (2001) Using clinical evidence. *BMJ.* **322**: 503–4.

Bass MJ, Dempsey B, McWhinney IR (1983) The natural history of headaches in family practice. In: *Proceedings of the Tenth World Conference of the World Organisation of National Colleges and Academies of General Practitioners*, Singapore.

Beate D, Skorpen J, Malterud K (1997) What did the doctor say and what did the patient do? Operational knowledge in clinical communication. *Fam Pract.* **4**: 376–81.

Benson J, Britten N (2002) Patients' decisions about whether or not to take antihypertensive drugs: a qualitative study. *BMJ.* **325**: 873–6.

Benson J, Britten N (2003) Patients' views about taking antihypertensive drugs: a questionnaire study. *BMJ.* **326**: 1314–15.

Borzak S, Ridker PM (1995) Discordance between meta-analysis and large-scale randomised controlled trials. *Ann Intern Med.* **123**: 873–7.

Bradley NCA, Sweeney KG, Waterfield M (1999) The health of their nation: how would citizens develop England's health strategy? *Br J Gen Pract.* **49**: 801–6.

Bryman A (1984) The debate about qualitative and quantitative methods: a question of method of epistemology? *Br J Sociol.* **35**: 75–92.

Budd J, Dawson S (1994) *Influencing Clinical Practice: implementation of research and development results. Report to North Thames Regional Health Authority.* Management School, Imperial College of Science, Technology and Medicine, London.

Byles JE, Hanrahan PF, Schofield MJ (1997) It would be good to know you're not alone: the health care needs of women with menstrual symptoms. *Fam Pract.* **14**: 249–54.

Cassell E (1991) *The Nature of Suffering and the Goal of Medicine.* Open University Press, Buckingham.

Chalmers I, Hetherington J, Newdick M *et al.* (1986) The Oxford Database of Perinatal Trials: developing a register of published reports of controlled trials. *Control Clin Trials.* **7**: 306–24.

Charlton IH, Charlton G, Broomfield J, Mulke MA (1991) Audit of the effect of a nurse-run asthma clinic on workload and patient morbidity in a general practice. *Br J Gen Pract.* **41**: 227–31.

Clarke N (2000) *Improving the Performance of Social Services* (PhD thesis). University of Exeter, Exeter.

Corney R (1995) Mental health services. In: Owens P, Carier J, Horder J (eds) *Interprofessional Issues in Community and Primary Health Care.* Macmillan, London.

Dalley B (1991) Beliefs and behaviour: professionals and the policy process. *J Ageing Stud.* **5**: 163–80.

Department of Health/Social Services Inspectorate (1989) *Working with Child Sexual Abuse: guidance for training social services staff.* HMSO, London.

Department of Health/Social Services Inspectorate (1991) *Care Management and Assessment: managers' guide.* HMSO, London.

Dixon AS (1986) There is a lot of it about: clinical strategies in family practice. *J R Coll Gen Pract.* **36**: 468–71.

Dudbridge SB, Stead J, Ward S, Antony M, Halpin DMG (1996) The Devon primary care asthma initiative: effects on morbidity. *Am J Respir Crit Care Med.* **53**: A868.

Early Breast Cancer Trialists' Collaborative Group (1992) Systematic treatment of early breast cancer by hormonal, cytotoxic or immune therapy: 133 randomised trials, involving 31 000 recurrences and 24 000 deaths among 75 000 women. *Lancet.* **339**: 71–85.

Egger M, Davey Smith G (1995) Misleading meta-analysis. *BMJ.* **310**: 752–4.

Egger M, Davey Smith G (1998) Meta-analysis: bias in location and selection of studies. *BMJ.* **316**: 61–6.

Egger M, Davey Smith G, Schneider M, Minder CE (1997) Bias in meta-analysis detected by a simple graphical test. *BMJ.* **315**: 629–34.

Evans M (2001) The medical body as philosophy's arena. *Theor Med Bioethics.* **1**: 17–23.

Feinstein A (1995) Meta-analysis: statistical alchemy for the twenty-first century. *J Clin Epidemiol.* **48**: 71–9.

Fibrinolytic Therapy Trialists' Group (1994) Indications for fibrinolytic therapy in suspected acute myocardial infarction: collaborative overview of early mortality and major morbidity results from all randomised trials of more than 1000 patients. *Lancet.* **343**: 311–22.

Fritsche L, Greenhalgh T, Falck-Ytter Y, Neumayer HH, Kunz R (2002) Do short courses in evidence-based medicine improve knowledge and skills? Validation of Berlin questionnaire before and after study of courses in evidence-based medicine. *BMJ.* **325**: 1338–41.

Gambetta D (1998) *Trust: making and breaking co-operative relations.* Blackwell, Oxford.

Glaser B (1992) *Emergence Versus Forcing Basics of Grounded Theory Analysis.* Sociology Press, CA.

Glaser B, Strauss A (1967) *The Discovery of Grounded Theory.* Aldine, Chicago.

Goffman E (1968) *Stigma: notes on the management of spoiled identity.* Penguin, Harmondsworth.

Good B (1994) *Medicine, Rationality and Experience.* Cambridge University Press, Cambridge.

Green J, Britten N (1998) Qualitative research and evidence-based medicine. *BMJ.* **316:** 1230–2.

Greenhalgh T, Hughes J, Humphrey C, Rogers S, Swinglehurst D, Martin P (2002) A comparative case study of two models of a clinical informaticist service. *BMJ.* **324:** 524–9.

Habermann-Little M (1991) Qualitative research methodologies: an overview. *J Neurosci Nurs.* **23:** 188–91.

Haynes RB (1993) Some problems in applying clinical evidence. In: Warren KS, Mosteller F (eds) *Doing More Good Than Harm: the evaluation of health care interventions.* Annals of New York Academy of Science, New York.

Haynes RB, Sackett D, Guyatt G, Cook D (1997) Transferring evidence from research to practice: overcoming barriers to application. *Evidence-Based Med.* **2:** 68–9.

Haynes RB, Devereaux PJ, Guyatt GH (2002) Physicians' and patients' choices in evidence-based medicine (editorial). *BMJ.* **324:** 1350.

Hilton S, Anderson HR, Sibbald B, Freeling P (1986) Controlled evaluation of the effects of patient-centred education on asthma morbidity in general practice. *Lancet.* **i:** 26–9.

Howitt A, Armstrong D (1999) Implementing evidence-based medicine in general practice: audit and qualitative study of antithrombotic treatment for atrial fibrillation. *BMJ.* **318:** 1324–7.

Hunter D (1993) It's not the knowing, it's the doing. *Health Serv J.* **7 October:** 21.

Hurwitz B (1996) Clinical guidelines and the law (editorial). *BMJ.* **311:** 1517–18.

Jacobson LD, Edwards ACK, Granier SK, Butler CC (1997) Evidence-based medicine and general practice. *Br J Gen Pract.* **47:** 449–52.

Jaeschke R, Guyatt G, Sackett DL for the Evidence-Based Medicine Working Group (1994) How to use an article about a diagnostic test. *JAMA.* **271:** 389–91.

Johnson M, Lakoff G (1980) *Metaphors We Live By.* University of Chicago Press, Chicago.

Jones I, Charlton IH, Middleton M, Preece WJ, Hill AP (1992) Targeting asthma care in general practice using a morbidity index. *BMJ.* **304:** 1353–6.

Jones K, Bain DJG, Middleton M, Mullee MA (1992) Correlates of asthma morbidity in primary care. *BMJ.* **304:** 361–5.

Jones R (1995) Why do qualitative research? (editorial). *BMJ.* **311:** 2.

Kellner R (1985) Functional somatic symptoms and hypochondriasis. *Arch Gen Psychiatry.* **42:** 821–33.

Kernick DP (2000) Muddling through in a parallel-track universe (letter). *Br J Gen Pract.* **50:** 65.

Kerridge I, Lowe M, Henry D (1998) Ethics and evidence-based medicine. *BMJ.* **316:** 1151–3.

Leary D (1994) *Metaphors in the History of Psychology.* Cambridge University Press, Cambridge.

Leedham I, Wistow G (1992) *Community Care and General Practitioners.* Nuffield Institute, Leeds.

Lehti A, Mattson B (2001) Health, attitude to care and pattern of attendance among gypsy women – a general practice perspective. *Fam Pract.* **18:** 445–8.

Lincoln YS, Guba EG (1985) *Naturalistic Enquiry.* Sage, Beverley Hills, CA.

Loxeley A (1997) *Collaboration in Health and Welfare: working with difference.* Jessica Kingsley Publishers, London.

Mabeck CE, Oleson F (1997) Metaphorically transmitted diseases. How do patients embody medical explanations? *Fam Pract.* **14:** 271–8.

McCormack J (1996) The death of the personal doctor. *Lancet.* **348:** 667–8.

McWhinney IR (1981) Problem solving and decision making. In: *An Introduction to Family Medicine.* Oxford University Press, Oxford.

McWhinney IR (1991) Primary care research in the next twenty years. In Norton P, Stewart M, Tudiver F, Bass M, Dunn E (eds) *Primary Care Research: traditional and innovative approaches.* Sage, Newbury Park, CA.

Maxwell JA (1992) Understanding and validity in qualitative research. *Harvard Educ Rev.* **62:** 279–300.

Mayer J, Piterman L (1999) The attitudes of Australian GPs to evidence-based medicine: a focus group study. *Fam Pract.* **16:** 627–32.

Melia KM (1996) Rediscovering Glaser. *Qual Health Res.* **6:** 368–78.

Miles HB, Huberman AM (1994) *Qualitative Data Analysis: an expanded sourcebook.* Sage Publications, Thousand Oaks, CA.

Mitchell D (2001) Implementing evidence in general practice. *BMJ Rapid Responses;* bmj.com/cgi/eletters/323/7231/1100.

Morgan DL (1988) *Focus Groups as Qualitative Research.* Sage Publications, London.

Morris NV, Abrahamson MJ, Strusser IT (1994) Adequacy of control of asthma in general practice. Is maximum peak expiratory flow rate a valid index of asthma severity? *Med J Aust.* **160:** 68–71.

Muir Gray JA (1999) Postmodern medicine. *Lancet.* **354:** 1550–3.

Murphy E, Mattison D (1992) Qualitative research and family practice: a marriage made in heaven? *Fam Pract.* **9:** 85–91.

O'Connor GT, Weiss ST (1994) Clinical and symptom measures. *Am J Respir Crit Care Med.* **149:** S21–8.

Ostergaard MS (1998) Childhood asthma: parents' perspective, a qualitative interview study. *Fam Pract.* **15:** 153–7.

Oxman A, Thomson MA, Davis DA, Haynes RB (1995) No magic bullets: a systematic review of 102 trials of interventions to improve professional practice. *J Can Med Assoc.* **153:** 1423–31.

Pereira Gray DJ (1995) Primary care and public health. *Health Hygiene.* **16:** 49–62.

Perrin K (2001) Better communication helps. *BMJ Rapid Responses;* bmj.com/cgi/eletters/323/7231/1100.

Potter J (1996) Discourse analysis and constructionist approaches: theoretical background. In: Richardson JT (ed.) *Handbook of Qualitative Research Methods in Psychology and Social Sciences.* BPS Books, Leicester.

Pringle M, Bradley CP, Carmichael CM, Wallace H, Moore A (1995) *Significant Event Audit.* Occasional Paper No. 70. Royal College of General Practitioners, London.

Rollnick S, Kinnersley P, Stott N (1993) Methods of helping patients with behaviour change. *BMJ.* **307:** 188–90.

Rudebeck CE (1992) General practice and a dialogue of clinical practice on symptoms, symptom presentations and bodily empathy. *Scand J Prim Health Care.* **Suppl. 1.**

Ryle G (1949) *The Concept of Mind.* Hutchinson, London.

Sackett DL (1992) A primer on the precision and accuracy of the clinical examination. *JAMA.* **267:** 2638–44.

Sackett DL, Richardson WS, Rosenberg W, Haynes RB (1997) *Evidence-Based Medicine: how to practise and teach EBM.* Churchill Livingstone, London.

Salinsky J (2001) Psychoanalysis and general practice: what did the Romans do for us? *Br J Gen Pract.* **51:** 506.

Schon DA (1995) *The Reflective Practitioner: how professionals think in action* (3e). Basic Books, King's Lynn.

Scott AJ (1977) Diagnostic accuracy would be improved by developing more categories of non-disease. *Med Hypotheses.* **3:** 135–7.

Secretary of State for Health (1996) *Promoting Clinical Effectiveness. A framework for action in and through the NHS.* NHS Executive, London.

Sheldon B (1994) Biological and social factors in mental disorders: implications for services. *Int J Psychiatry.* **40:** 87–105.

Silverman HA (ed.) (1980) *Piaget, Philosophy and the Human Sciences.* Northwestern University Press, Evanston, IL.

Silverman WA, Altman DG (1996) Patients' preferences and randomised trials. *Lancet.* **347:** 171–4.

Skelton JR, Hobbs EDR (1999) Concordancing: use of language-based research in medical communication. *Lancet.* **353:** 108–11.

Skelton J, Hobbs FDR (1999) Descriptive study of cooperative language in primary care consultations by male and female doctors. *BMJ.* **318:** 576–9.

Stagnaro S (2001) The complex relations between GPs and evidence. *BMJ Rapid Responses;* bmj.com/cgi/eletters/323/7231/1100.

Stern PN (1994) Eroding grounded theory. In: Morse JM (ed.) *Critical Issues in Qualitative Research Methods.* Sage Publications, Thousand Oaks, CA.

Strauss A (1978) *Negotiations: varieties, contexts, processes and social order.* Jossey-Bass, San Francisco, CA.

Strauss A, Corbin J (1990) *The Basics of Qualitative Research-Grounded Theory Procedures and Techniques.* Sage, Newbury Park, CA.

Strauss SE, Sackett DL (1998) Using research findings in clinical practice. *BMJ.* **317:** 339–42.

Sweeney G, Sweeney K, Greco M, Stead J (2002) Softly softly – the way forward. A qualitative study of the first year of implementing clinical governance in primary care. *Prim Health Care Res Dev.* **3:** 53–64.

Sweeney K (1996) *The use of focus in groups to assess consumers' views on miscarriage and minor surgery* (MPhil thesis). University of Exeter, Exeter.

Teo KK, Yusuf S, Colling R *et al.* (1991) Effects of intravenous magnesium in suspected acute myocardial infarction: overview of randomised trials. *BMJ.* **303:** 1499–503.

Thomas KB (1974) Temporarily dependent patients in general practice. *BMJ.* **i:** 59–65.

Thompson SG, Pocock SJ (1991) Can meta-analysis be trusted? *Lancet.* **338:** 1127–30.

Tomlin Z, Humphrey C, Rogers S (1999) General practitioners' perceptions of effective health care. *BMJ.* **318:** 1532–5.

Toulmin S (1993) Knowledge in the practice of medicine: clinical judgment and historical reconstruction. In: Delkeshamp-Hayes C, Gardell Cutter MAG (eds) *Science, Technology and the Art of Medicine. European–American dialogues.* Kluwer, Dordrecht.

Turner-Warwick M (1989) Nocturnal asthma: a study in general practice. *J R Coll Gen Pract.* **39:** 239–43.

Veldhuis M, Wigersma L, Okkes I (1998) Deliberate departures from good general practice: a study of motives among Dutch general practitioners. *Br J Gen Pract.* **48:** 1833–6.

Wakefield AJ, Murch SH, Anthony A *et al.* (1998) Ileal lymphoid nodular hyperplasia, non-specific colitis, and pervasive developmental disorder in children. *Lancet.* **351:** 637–41.

Wells S (2001) Knowledge management, a balanced approach. *BMJ Rapid Responses;* bmj.com/cgi/eletters/323/7231/1100.

West RR (1993) A look at the statistical overview (or meta-analysis). *J R Coll Physicians Lond.* **27:** 111–15.

Westcott R, Sweeney G, Stead J (2000) Significant event audit in practice: a preliminary study. *Fam Pract.* **17:** 173–9.

Willis J (1995) *The Paradox of Progress.* Radcliffe Medical Press, Oxford.

Workman S (2001) It appears evidence-based practice is a skill which must be taught. *BMJ Rapid Responses;* bmj.com.

Index